PANACEA ON EARTH
The three most powerful pages that can change your Life

Yes That's right. The three pages that you have just started reading have the potential to change your life forever. For I am going to reveal to you the **Panacea** on earth. It will change the way you think about health and then you'll never be required to visit any hospital or health centre to cure dreaded diseases.

It had been in use since ages. One can find its mention and use in the pages of mythology and world history. Let me give some of the endorsees of this humble little secret.

1) **Lord Ganesha** once swallowed a mighty demon and developed a burning sensation in his stomach. No God or doctor all over the cosmos could relieve him from his burning pain. Then 8800 sages gave him this food that we are talking about & he got immediate relief.

2) **Jesus Christ** asked his men and mankind to take this food to cure themselves of any disease.

3) This food was taken by **Egyptian Kings** and soldiers of **Mesopotamian** civilization to keep themselves healthy.

4) **Shushruta** who wrote "Shushruta Samhita" and is known as 'father of Surgery', used this to heal the injuries and wounds of his patients.

5) It was used during the reign of **Chandragupta Maurya** to heal and cure wounds and injuries.

6) The great Arab-traveler **Ibn–e-battuta** or Hajji Abu-Abdulla Muhammad was a Moroccan. He is known for his fascinating travels spanning thirty years. He started his journey at the age of twenty-one (1325) and ended it in 1355. During his travel in 1348, when he was in

Damascus Syria ,he got sick. That time, the whole world was under a pandemic called Bubonic Plague, also known as Black-Death. It was the most devastating pandemic in human History. Ibn-e-Battuta too caught this plague. One of his professors helped him to get cured. This professor gave him the juice of this wonder food and other concoctions. He was back on his foot soon and left for India.

7) **Babylonian King Nebuchadnezzar II,** who built 'Hanging Garden of Babylon' to please his homesick wife Amytis of Media, once got very sick and lost his mental balance. He was sick for seven long years. Finally he got cured consuming fruits, vegetables and herbs and this food.

This Humble little panacea on Earth is nothing else but, **"WHEATGRASS"**

The famous inventor of Electric Bulb, **Thomas Alva Edison** also quoted, "until man duplicates a blade of grass, nature can laugh at his so called scientific knowledge".

Intuitive intelligence of cats, dogs and other carnivores, tells them to nibble on grass whenever they fall sick.

So a new question popping up in your mind would be:-

How Wheatgrass Heals?

Here I would like to shift your focus from mythology and history towards concrete facts and logic.

Wheatgrass helps in healing by:

1.Restoring the damaged neurons.

2. Restoring the organ damage.

3. Behaviour modification.

4. Restoring the intuitive intelligence.

5. Complete mind–body cleansing.

6. Optimzing the hormonal balance.

And to complete the answer I will tell you

Why Wheatgrass Heals?

Because it contains:

1. Power of sunlight in condensed form.

2. All the 92 nutrients out of 102 nutients in the appropriate ratio as needed by human body for perfect balance.

3. Mind–body–soul alignment through perfect vibrational energy.

Truly said, by Hippocrates, the father of modern medicine, "Not the Doctor, but Nature Heals".

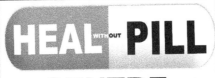

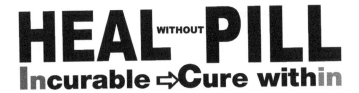

HEAL WITHOUT PILL
Incurable ➪ Cure within

Dr. Biswaroop Roy Chowdhury

(Multiple Guinness World Records Holder)

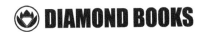
DIAMOND BOOKS

Published by:

🌸 **Diamond Pocket Books Pvt. Ltd.**
X-30, Okhla Industrial Area
Phase-II, New Delhi-20
Tel : 011-40712200
E-mail : sales@dpb.in   website : www.dpb.in

Graphics Designer   : Shankar Singh Koranga
Research & Development : Pratiksha Vats, Rachna Sharma
Proof Reading   : Rita Sharma, Anupama Sharma
Cartoonist   : Rahul, Amit, Manjeet

DEDICATION

Dedicated to my parents who have
been the source of inspiration for
my creative writing

DISCLAIMER

This book is designed to provide information about the subject matter covered. While all attempts have been made to verify information provided in this publication, neither the author nor the publisher assumes any responsibility for errors, omissions or contrary interpretation of the subject matter.

The purchaser or reader of this publication assumes responsibility for the use of these materials and information. The author and publisher assume no responsibility or liability whatsoever on behalf of any purchaser or reader of these materials.

The purpose of this workbook is to educate. Any perceived slight to specific individual or organization is unintentional.

This book is the way to make better-educated decisions, to find the root cause of life's challenges and show ways to eliminate these causes. It also is intended to help you to establish your personal level of optimum health in the shortest amount of time.

CONTENT

CHAPTER -ONE

HOW TO READ THIS BOOK

Welcome to the world of nature to which each and every creature of this planet is close, except the human being. This book will work as a guide to recreate that lost bond with the nature and solve every health problem, in the nature's way.

To get the most out of this book, try to read the book in order. Do not skip any chapter. I would suggest you to read the book in parts (divide it in 10 parts) rather than reading it in one go. Read one part a day and try to associate it with your day to day activities.

Your quest and craving for a finer and superior health will be the foremost factor to extract and gain the maximum from the book.

Reading merely for leisure will be of little use. Your commitment, yearning, hunger and dedication towards yourself and religious implementation of the methods given in following pages will indubitably transform your health.

Now, let's be nostalgic...and look back over past ten years... So what did you find! Were there times when a 'different' decision would have made your life radically different from today? *'The Road Not Taken'* kind of situation.... a predicament that could have made your life better or even worse! Say... you made a decision for your career or job and that changed your life or you missed the shot... or perhaps you decided to get married (wow)or divorced (Opps). You might have purchased an audio tape, a book or attended a seminar or met somebody, who eventually changed your belief system and actions for ever. May be you decided to start exercising or to give up or you decided to quit smoking...

whatever in fact, happens in your life –either when you are 'ecstatic' 'thrilled' or 'challenged' by this or that factor........your reaction, your response– all began with a 'decision' a 'resolution'. I strongly believe that it is in that moment, when your destiny is shaped and takes its own course.

Your today's decision to strictly follow the system given in the book will pave your way to a 'Superior' Health forever.

CHAPTER -TWO

MEDICINE: BOON OR BANE

According to 'News Week' August 22-29, 2011 issue "One word that will save your life".

Yes! In today's world of scientific discoveries and advancement and medical health care facilities, one word that will save you is **"No"**...No to any kind of medical tests and treatments. The article further elaborates citing the example of Dr Rita Redberg, who is a professor of medicine at the University of California, San Francisco and Editor of prestigious Archives of Internal

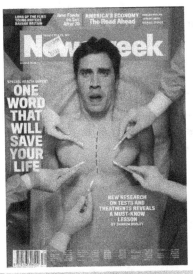

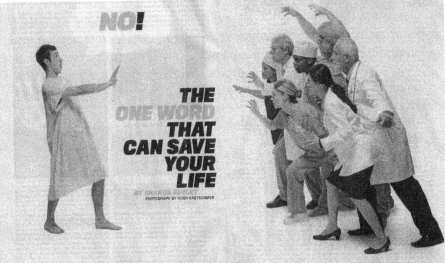

THE OMNIPRESENT MRI, NEW RRESEARCH SHOWS HOW SOME COMMON TESTS AND PROCEDURES AREN'T JUST EXPENSIVE, BUT CAN DO MORE HARM THAN GOOD.

Medicines. She has no intention of having a screening mammogram done to detect the presence of breast tumor, if any, even though her 50th birthday has come and gone. But Dr. Redberg says, these tests falsely detect positive tumors that might regress on their own and there is little evidence that these tests save lives. Sometimes, the so called medical advances and health care system make the matter worse. There are many areas of medicine where not testing, not imaging and not treating actually result in better health and conversely more healthcare can harm the health. Most of us wouldn't think twice if our doctor offered a test that has the power to expose a lurking tumor or a clogged artery, or a heart arrhythmia . Better to know and get treated than to take risks .In fact, for many otherwise healthy people, tests often lead to more tests, which can lead to interventions based on a possible problem that may have gone away on its own or ultimately proved harmless. Some of the most disturbing examples involve cardiology. The studies done for this compared invasive procedure including angioplasty. Every study found that the surgical procedure didn't improve survival rates or quality of life more than the non-invasive treatment including drugs, exercise and healthy diet. It turns out that big blockages that show up on CT scans and other imaging, that were long believed to be causing heart –attack usually don't cause them. But treating these blockages can! This is because when you try to clean up this blockage through surgery, a whole lot of debris after cleaning gets into the blood vessels and that may trigger a heart attack or stroke. There is a long standing fallacy among physicians that if you find something different from what you perceive normal. Then it must be the cause of the problem. Today's comprehensive blood tests measure 15 or so enzymes, proteins, lipids and the like. Yet by chance, if you test for 20 things, something will fall outside the bounds of normal, often, due to simple lab errors.

Many doctors don't seem to be getting the message about useless and harmful health care. Several large studies, including the Occluded Artery Trial in 2006 have shown that inserting a stent to prop open a blocked artery more than 24 hrs after a heart attack does not improve survival rates or reduce the risk of another coronary block at a rate of 100,000 a year.

They are killing more people than they are saving with these procedures. Its as simple as that.

Another term that is an extension of these tests and treatment is **"Disease Mongering"** .There is a whole lot of money that can be made from healthy people, if they are made to believe that they are sick. Health industry have "medicalized" the idea of well being, promoting the idea that everyone has something wrong with him/her. Previously 'fat and happy' is now considered being 'obese and unhealthy'. The medical industry in order to generate more profits, medicalizes normal life experiences by turning every emotion, behaviour, habit and mood into a disease requiring medical or chemical treatments.

In other words disease mongering is the selling of sickness that widens the boundaries of illness and grows the market for pharmaceutical companies. The companies fund free disease-awareness campaigns which are more often designed to sell medicines/drugs than to illuminate, inform or educate people about the prevention of illness and the maintenance of health. The strategy is to convince as many people as possible that they have medical conditions that require long term drug treatment.

A central disease mongering tactic is to attach complex, scientific sounding names to minor easily curable conditions.
For example:
1) Occasional heartburn becomes Gastro- Esophageal Reflux Disease or GERD.
2) Impotence becomes "Erectile Dysfunction"or ED.
3) Premenstrual tension becomes "Premenstrual Dysphoric Disorder or PMDD.
4) Shyness becomes "Social Anxiety Disorder " or SAD.
5) Fidgeting legs becomes "Restless Leg Syndrome" or RLS.

So what should be done ! The answers is to resort to the best medicine. i.e modification in diet, exercise or simple stress reduction techniques or to simply wait, give the body's own healing mechanism a chance to find equilibrium to get on with our lives.

On the other hand we cannot deny that millions of patients throughout the world benefit each year from the life saving and life enhancing drugs. The contribution of science and technology over the past few centuries have been immense, especially during $18^{th}, 19^{th}$ & 20th century.

The works of Isaac Newton, Robert Boyle and Robert Hooke, William Harvey signaled the beginning of modern scientific medicine. The most significant medical breakthrough has been the discovery and development of antibiotics. Once incurable diseases like cholera, typhoid and plague have either been eradicated or have been tackled effectively.

The other huge advantage is **vaccination** .Small Pox, Plague, Diphtheria, Whooping Cough, Tuberculosis, Tetanus and Yellow Fever, which were once considered as potential killers have been eradicated through immunization and vaccination.

Polio is next on list. WHO hopes to eradicate it within the next few years.

The numbers of different organs that can be replaced in human is extra ordinary. Lungs, Heart, Kidneys, Cornea, Liver, Pancreas, Skin, Bone-marrow & even entire bones are harvested from living or dead donors and swapped for diseased organs.

Latest development is the stem cell therapy. Scientists believe that stem cell therapy can change the face of human diseases and alleviate suffering .Stem cells (derived) from bone marrow in adults and umbilical cord in infants have the potential to regenerate the damaged or diseased organs/areas of the body.

Diseases that were once fatal have either diminished or disappeared. The major advances in medical science have changed societies and its expectations greatly.

CHAPTER -THREE

OUR BODY-THE BEST MANAGER OF ITS BIOCHEMISTRY

Our body contains some *50 trillion* cells, all working like miniature chemical factories and each of them has a certain working pathway. These pathways form a complicated *network*.

The biochemical processes that maintain our bodies are much more complex than anyone ever realized. In just one tiny cell (quite invisible to the naked eye) a plan of all the chemical interactions would look like an extremely complex three dimensional television circuit diagram. When we eat badly in ways that are discordant with the blueprint of the cells, it disrupts the body's micro management.

There are many manifestations of so-called food and disease connections. One of the less familiar is the food and arthritis connection. This is a disease that is becoming widespread under the influence of poor dietary practices. One of these is the faulty consumption of essential fatty acids.

Today's diet is overbalanced in favor of linoleic acid – mostly corn oil, sunflower oil, and peanut oil. Linoleic acid is converted into a series of different hormones which can be either *beneficial* or *harmful*. And that depends on the intake of other dietary factors.

The sample hormone cascade on next page shows how linoleic acid is transformed into hormones. The transformation into hormones is blocked if the enzyme Delta 6 Desaturase is not formed which in turn is controlled by bad carbohydrates and insulin. But there is another enzyme Delta 5 Desaturase, the presence of this enzyme *decides which way* the hormonal transformation will go i.e. either *Good* or *bad* messages to the

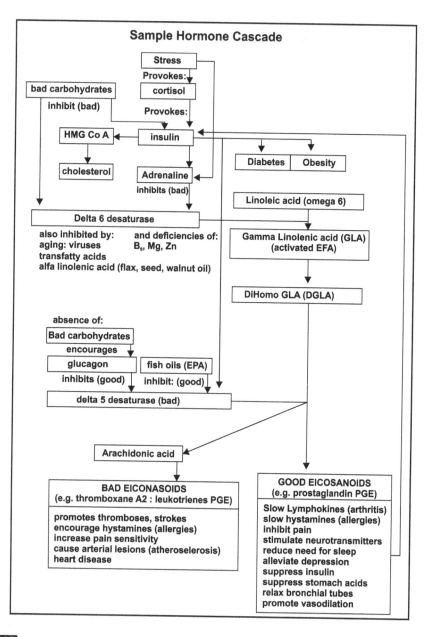

Sample Hormone Cascade

Stress
Provokes:
cortisol
Provokes:

bad carbohydrates
inhibit (bad)

HMG Co A

cholesterol

insulin

Adrenaline
inhibits (bad)

Diabetes | Obesity

Linoleic acid (omega 6)

Delta 6 desaturase

also inhibited by: and deficiencies of:
aging: viruses B_6, Mg, Zn
transfatty acids
alfa linolenic acid (flax, seed, walnut oil)

Gamma Linolenic acid (GLA)
(activated EFA)

DiHomo GLA (DGLA)

absence of:
Bad carbohydrates
encourages
glucagon   fish oils (EPA)
inhibits (good)   inhibit: (good)

delta 5 desaturase (bad)

Arachidonic acid

BAD EICONASOIDS
(e.g. thromboxane A2 : leukotrienes PGE)

promotes thromboses, strokes
encourage hystamines (allergies)
increase pain sensitivity
cause arterial lesions (atheroselerosis)
heart disease

GOOD EICOSANOIDS
(e.g. prostaglandin PGE)

Slow Lymphokines (arthritis)
slow hystamines (allergies)
inhibit pain
stimulate neurotransmitters
reduce need for sleep
alleviate depression
suppress insulin
suppress stomach acids
relax bronchial tubes
promote vasodilation

body's cells. Some people have heard that arthritis can be helped by the consumption of GLA (Gamma Linoleic acid). This is present in Evening Primrose Oil. But taking GLA does not determine what the body is going to do with it. It could still be turned into compounds, by the Delta 5 Desaturase, that *aggravate* arthritis rather than alleviate it. It all depends what other things you are taking in your diet. It is also known as the 'Law of Unintended Consequences'.

To make the complexity of our body biochemistry more clear lets take another example. Our understanding of vitamins and minerals has improved dramatically. We all know these micro nutrients play a crucial role in maintaining good health and keeping diseases at bay. To ensure a balanced intake of these vitamins and minerals we often resort to vitamin supplements which can be easily bought from any chemist shop. The most common vitamin supplement consumed all over the world today is Vitamin C. It is known to fight cancer and other infectious diseases. But these vitamins and minerals do not work alone. They have a direct or indirect impact on the metabolism and absorption of other vitamins and minerals too. For example the vitamin C supplement that we consume, boosts our immunity on one hand but increases the absorption of iron in our body, on the other. This may lead to the over absorption of iron and the result would be iron toxicity.
Excessive Iron then interferes with zinc and copper metabolism, which are needed to maintain the integrity of the bone joints. Excessive iron antagonizes chromium needed for insulin transport. Iron, in excess, by causing a zinc deficiency, results in diabetes. Zinc is needed for insulin production. Iron buildup in the pancreas results in pancreatic damage.

A high protein diet, caffeine from coffee, carbonated beverages, alcohol, and antacids can diminish calcium levels in our body. An excessive intake of Calcium will reduce our body's level of Magnesium. Magnesium on the other hand is necessary for Calcium and Vitamin C metabolism. Iron, high

INTER-RELATIONSHIP BETWEEN VARIOUS DIETERY FACTORS

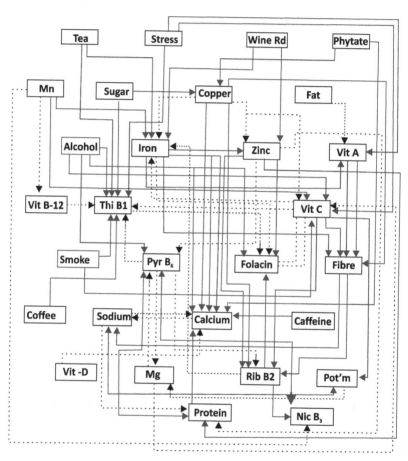

1. Dotted lines represent positive impact.
2. Dark lines represent negative/inhibitory impact.

calcium diets and magnesium inhibit manganese absorption in our body which is needed for protein and fat metabolism...Similarly, stress at work, tea, coffee, sugar, alcohol and wine also play a major role in absorption and interaction among various dietary factors.

The figure on page 20 shows the intricate inter-relationship of various minerals, vitamins and other factors in the diet. Dark lines indicate inhibitory or restrictive impact whereas dotted lines represent positive and favorable impact and interactions among dietary nutrients.

The big question that now arises is...How can one find the right balance! The answer is....it is IMPOSSIBLE.

The message is, it is impossible to micro manage these processes. But our own bodies are incredibly well endowed with their own self management mechanisms.

Our own body is the best manager of its biochemistry

It means we have to return to the pattern of eating to which our bodies have been adapted over millions of years - to that eaten by our prehistoric forebearers. It is a way of eating which is in *harmony* with the way our bodies have evolved. It is *Natural*.

CHAPTER -FOUR

WHATEVER DISEASE YOU MAY BE SUFFERING FROM YOU WILL BE HEALED

I don't know who you are and which disease you are suffering from? But I can tell you, with complete conviction and assurance that even if it is 3rd stage of cancer or advanced diabetes you can reclaim your health. Surprised!!! This book, in 8 easy steps will guide you to build your own Super Specialty Home Hospital in less than ₹ 10,000/- in just one week, which can help you to treat diseases from common cold to chronic constipation, from mild acidity to severe arthritis.

Be your own doctor and never fall sick again...

CHAPTER -FIVE

WHY DO WE GET A DISEASE?
(Part-I)

We are designed and created by the nature not to be diseased, but to live a healthy life of not less than150 years, as our ancestors used to live. It happens only, when we break the rule of Nature, we fall sick and become prone to an ailment.

Why do we get a disease. It depends chiefly on two significant factors:

1) What do we eat?

2) What do we think?

Let's understand the 1st factor "What do we eat?"

Try to recall *November 26, 2008*, Mumbai was attacked by terrorists, entire world stood shocked, stunned and flabbergasted, when terrorists ransacked, the beautiful Hotel 'Taj' and fired indiscriminately at people in the hotel, smashed up the beautiful hotel and even set a part of it on fire. Thus causing an irreparable damage to the beauty and the integrity of *'Amachi Mumbai'*.

Now, co-relate yourself with *the Hotel Taj* , visualize terrorists as some of the detrimental injurious, deceiving food items, which you unsuspectingly allow to enter into your body, analogous to the guards of Taj Hotel, who could not sense the true identity and allowed the terrorists to enter inside. Terrorists must have disguised themselves as elegant, sophisticated and genuine guests.

Let's meet the 'terrorists' hidden in your food 'carte du jour' (menu) .....

Let's contemplate how most of us start a normal day... We refuse to open our eyes and come out of bed untill served a 'bed tea'. Another name you can give to your bed tea is a 'slow poison'. Take a closer look...

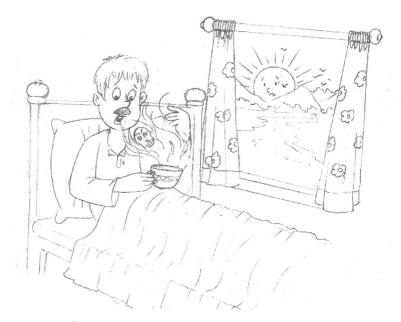

Dawn of the Day with Slow Poison , 'Tea'.

Just give a second, note what the ingredients of your tea are

a little milk + refined sugar + tea leaves and water.

Terrorist No. 1 SUGAR:

Sugar is just like Osama Bin Laden, very adamant, very inquisitive, very hard-hitting and above all penetrating. It can enter even the strongest, the toughest and the remotest organ and can pierce even through the fattest cell membrane of the body and can cause more than...can you believe it... 150 diseases. Name a disease and literally 'Mr. Sugar' plays a vital role in "accomplishing" that disease.

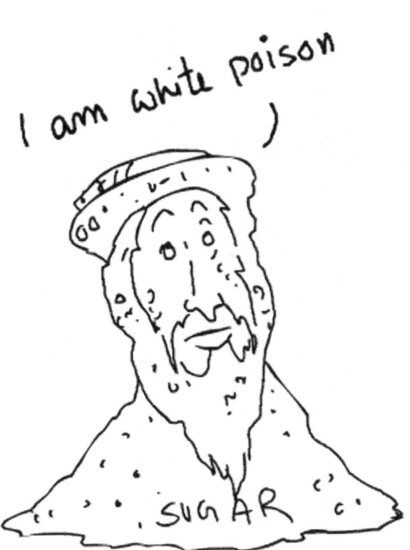

'Refined Sugar', A Hard Hitting White Poison Is Associated With A Long List Of Health Problems.

It so happens because loads of calcium, sodium, potassium and magnesium is required to digest the refined sugar and they have to be taken from the various parts of the body. Consequently body falls short of these vital elements and the micronutrients. This results in everything from Osteoporosis to the failure of effective excretion of poisonous residues and wastes.

We can call refined sugar a 'sweet poison'. Due to space restriction I am unable to supply you with the long list of diseases, where sugar plays a pivotal role, as it will take not less than 50 pages. Pointless to mention, not only tea but any food item, having sugar as an important ingredient like chocolates, candies, sweets, cold drinks, can result in a diseased body. I feel extremely pained to discover that these are the main food items, 'Hot favourites' among children.

Some may raise a doubt here and argue that sugar plays an important role in the growth and development of the body, but dear friends.....remember it is sugar in its natural form as in fruits, honey etc. not the 'refined sugar'.

Terrorist No. 2 Milk:

1. Nature has bestowed mammals to feed their young ones with milk. Every mammal's milk is intended and meant for the development of its young ones only. Milk produced by a species is not suitable for the other species'. Except humans, no animal drinks the milk of any other animal.

2. I do agree that milk is wholly required during the infancy, when the infant is not able to take any other solid or liquid food, but milk is not meant for the lifelong use; no animal except human being continues to drink the milk lifetime.

I propose to *Be A Vegan* because biologically speaking human body is not designed rather it is incapable to digest cow's or even buffalo's milk. During infancy, body has certain enzymes which help in the digestion of milk but with age those enzymes become inactive, as a result some components of milk get glued to various parts of the digestive system, resulting in overall blockage of the most of the systems in our body and prevents the absorbtion of the nutrients in the body.

Co-relate your city with sewage system. What if, it gets blocked. The 'wastes' will not be drained out and end up in blocking your toilet ...gradually bathroom and eventually the complete house. Remember one of the strongest glue (Elmer's glue) in the world is made from the cow's milk.

Terrorist No. 3 Caffeine:

Its characteristics match more like a crooked politician, who promises 'common man' to provide with all luxuries, ironically which originally belonged to common man only.

Most of us relish a cup (or a big Mug) of tea with a belief that it will give us instant energy, alertness and refreshness. Actually, what happens is exactly the reverse, it is not the energy of the Caffeine but the 'stolen' energy from the emergency reserves of the body. To compensate for this lost energy, body has to work harder obviously resulting in some serious damages and disorders. That is why, after a cup of coffee, the *initial high* is followed by a series of tiredness and fatigue. So remember this refreshing cup may later on bring a few little 'surprises' for you, in the forms of diabetes, kidney and liver damage etc.

Like those unsuspecting guards, who allowed terrorists in the hotel, believing them to be genuine guests, but turned out to be criminals. Similarly throughout the day, we eat a lot of food items believing, once it is inside the body, it will help in the growth and maintenance of the body, on the contrary it comes out to be a deadly poison. Let's uncover them bit by bit.

Terrorist No. 4 Refined Cereal:

White flour and polished rice are the two most widely used refined cereals in our day to day food. In white flour, the outer husk of the wheat and bran is removed, while in polished rice ,the outer brown husk is removed during refining. In both cases husks are the major source of vitamins, minerals and fibers. Common white flour preparations include white bread, naan, romali roti, pizza, biscuit, cake, noodles etc. Common polished rice delicacies are pullao, biryani, plain fried rice and dosa etc.

Vitamin-B Deficiency: Vitamin B is necessary for the digestion and assimilation of rice and flour. None of the Vitamin-Bs is present in refined cereals. Hence for absorption and assimilation, the Vitamin-B is stolen from nerves, muscles, liver, kidney, stomach, heart, skin, eyes, blood etc. leaving these organs wanting in Vitamin-B. Imagine you are constantly withdrawing from your account, but not depositing any money. Surely one day you will be penniless. The more these refined foods are taken in, more is the amount of Vitamin-B stolen from the various organs of the body. We thus suffer from nervous irritability, digestive disorders, tiredness, poor eyesight, anemia, heart trouble, muscular diseases etc.

Terrorist No. 5 Table- Salt:

Small amount of salt (sodium ions) is needed to maintain a good health especially for neurons. The salt in its natural form which is found in vegetables like potatoes, onions, tomatoes etc. is sufficient to keep us healthy.

Table Salt is a strongly ionic bonded, inorganic compound and resists being separated into the sodium and chloride which are usable by the body. Hence it doesn't replenish the sodium needs of the body. Imagine you are gifted a nice pair of shoes, but with the laces tied to each other permanently. Will it be of any use! The salt present in fruits and vegetables is organic in nature and loosely covalently bonded and thus can be easily separated and utilized by the body.

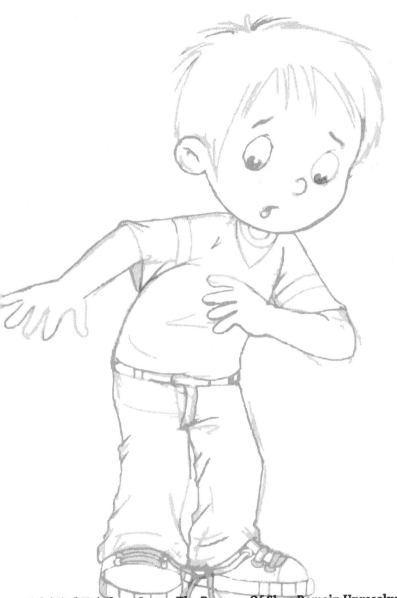

With 'Tied Up' Shoes Laces, The Purpose Of Shoe Remain Unresolved.
Same Way, Strongly 'Ionic Bonded' Table Salt Remains Unused By The Body.

Terrorist No. 6 Fried Food:

The frying and prolonged heating of food leads to the formation of FREE RADICALS. A free radical is a molecule that has lost one electron and has become highly imbalanced. It restores its balance by stealing a vital electron from other molecules.

Just like a chappal chor (shoe thief). Imagine people entering inside a temple, leaving their slippers outside, but when a person comes out of the temple he finds only one of the slipper of the pair. To complete the pair, he steals other person's one of the slipper. The next person on discovering that he has lost one of the slippers, decides to steal some other person's one slipper and the whole range of vicious chain reaction starts. Free radicals are just like these thieves that start the chain reaction of stealing electrons from other molecules, thus resulting in a major imbalance in the system. Consumption of fried food is an open invitation to all kinds of diseases.

Just think about burgers, pizzas, chips, patties and french fries. It is frozen, deep fried and micro-waved. Exposure to micro-wave emission has a negative effect on the general biological welfare of humans, i.e it forms cancer causing free radicals. I will not give such food even to my dog. It is no better than a pile of garbage, just fit for vulture. Micro-wave's exposure causes significant decrease in the nutritive value. Because of unnatural processing, these foods are devoid of enzymes; so it becomes very difficult for the digestive system to digest such food items and so most of the food remains suitable for the excretion as shit / faeces and also the processing makes the food fibreless.

Fibers in our intestinal track work like a broom helping the faecal matter to push through the colon for excretion, due to lack of fibers in our food items ,the faecal matter stays in the form of garbage and get dumped for long time inside the colon.

To imagine the condition of the colon, try imagining yourself given a

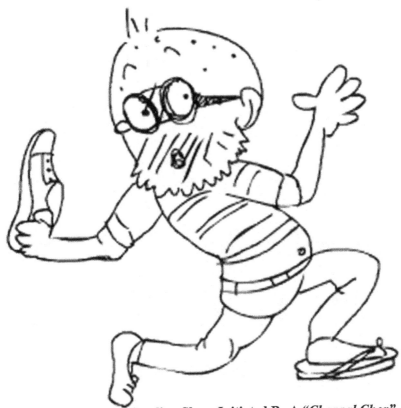

'Chain Reaction' Of Stealing Shoes Initiated By A "Chappal Chor"
Is Similar To The One Initiated By 'Free Radicals' Causing Imbalance
In The System.

punishment of standing inside the dirtiest garbage site of your city for hours. Remember colon is connected to all the organs of the body through nerves (Refer page no. 32 & 33) even to the eyeballs. Many times severe headache, nausea and fatigue are caused directly from the colon, burdened with immovable faeces in the colon gifted by your beloved burgers, pizzas, french fries and other fast food items.

The Pizza Challenge: Eat pizza in breakfast, lunch and dinner straight

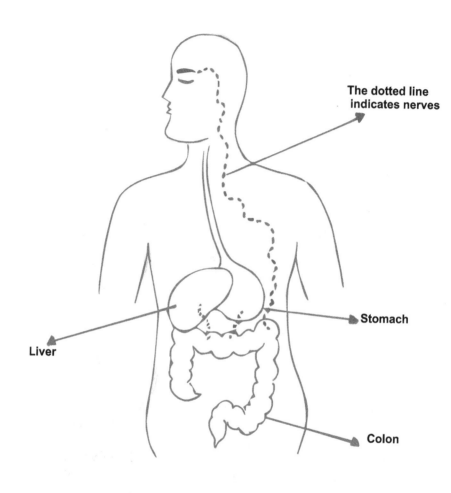

The dotted line indicates nerves

Stomach

Liver

Colon

**Picture Showing Connection of Colon
With Other Organs Through Nerves**

for just only one month and the free offer you will get is... a walking museum of diseases. So next time before you gobble down a burger or a pizza, visualize yourself sitting inside the worst smelling sewage garbage of the world.

Shocking Facts about Fast Foods:

Fact I : 99% of the fast foods including from McDonald, KFC and Subway contain taste enhancing agent called MSG, which is responsible for more than 90% diseases including cancer, heart attack, diabetes, migraine etc.

Fact II: Owner of Baskin Robbins died by eating his own ice-cream.

Fact III: McDonald themselves accepted that their food is harmful for health.

Fact IV: Two litres of soft drink if taken in one go can lead to choking and may cause even death.

Fact V: Aspartine is an artificial low calorie sweetener also called as taste enhancer. It is commonly included in most of the fast foods and soft drinks, more over it is approximately 200 times sweeter than sugar and causes a number of mental illnesses. Neuroscience says, sometimes the symptoms appear only after 90% of the neurons of a particular area of the brain are dead.

Fact V1: To neutralize the ill effects of a glass of soft drink, human body needs 32 glasses of water intake.

PART I: Enjoying Life Full With Fast Food For Few Years.

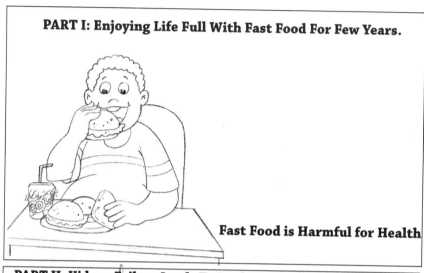

Fast Food is Harmful for Health

PART II: Kidney Failure Leads To Replacement Of Donar Kidney.

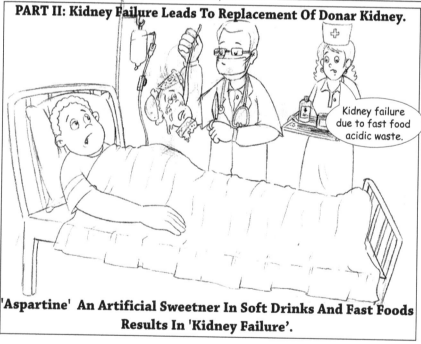

Kidney failure due to fast food acidic waste.

'Aspartine' An Artificial Sweetner In Soft Drinks And Fast Foods Results In 'Kidney Failure'.

CHAPTER -SIX

MORE ON FAST FOOD: AN EYE OPENER

Birthday party of a six year old........
All friends invited for the party......
Two tables lay with different carte du jour...........

On one table fruits, sprouts, vegetable salad, fresh fruit juice, and home made dinner nicely decorated with parsley, green coriander and freshly squeezed lemon juice is served, on the other burgers, pizzas, french-fries, noodles, chips, chocolates, cold drinks are served. Now let the children have the food of their choice.

What do you think would their choice be!

The choice is obvious...Fast food!

We often blame our kids for having an affinity towards eating out, for preferring fast food over home made food.

What make these kids incline towards such food! Why do they like it so much!

The reason is quite obvious. These fast foods win over your home made food not because they are nutritious. They triumph because they are tastier and spicier.

Here I am not referring to traditional spices but the artificial tastemakers, flavours and a myriad variety of salts and chemicals used in them.

These chemicals serve two purposes- one augments taste/flavor of a low quality food, as it masks the real taste of the food. Secondly, but very important commercially, it increases their shelf life. Children tend to develop a sort of addiction for them as little they know about the chemicals being added. This food not only enslaves their taste buds but also interferes with their brain and thus I am not wrong in using the word. It's ADDICTIVE! And addiction of anything is detrimental...

Trust me or try it...if these chemicals mixed with handful of soil and given to children they will eat it happily and surprisingly will find it equally delicious and yummy... That's what these chemicals (Neurotoxins or Excitotoxins) do... enhance Flavors' and excite the brain ultimately damaging it.

These Neurotoxins or Excitotoxins (MSG and Aspartame)are amino acids that serve as neurotransmitters in the brain. The nervous system needs amino acid neurotransmitters to operate. But when the dose is too high or builds from excessive daily intake, these amino acids cross the blood brain barrier and excite the neurons of brain cells to a point of absolute exhaustion. Then those brain neurons eventually die.

MSG (Mono Sodium Glutamate):

Monosodium glutamate, also known as sodium glutamate and MSG, is a sodium salt of glutamic acid, a naturally occurring non-essential amino acid. It is used as a food additive and is commonly marketed as a flavour enhancer.

MSG(Use in Cooking):

MSG is used extensively in Japanese cooking, where it is sold under the brand name Ajinomoto, and in Chinese restaurants, which use it to "beef up" dishes. Traditional cooking actually uses little meat and lots of vegetables, and MSG makes it more satisfyingly meaty. MSG use, however, is not confined to Asian Cuisine. Ajinomoto is a very popular seasoning in the world. Throughout the food industry, MSG is an increasingly popular way to add flavor to packaged foods as well as fast foods such as burgers, pizzas, french-fries, soups, sauces, seasonings, and instant snacks, chips, cold drinks, fruit juices, energy drinks.

Foods Containing MSG and Hidden Sources of MSG

MSG is used around the globe in soups and broths, sauces, gravies, and flavoring and spice blends. MSG is also present in a variety of processed foods such as canned and frozen meats, fish, poultry, vegetables, and ready-to-eat food plates, dressings, ketchup, mayonnaise, soy sauce, sausages, snacks, some processed cheese, soup powders for instant noodles, etc.

MSG usage is sometimes "hidden" in food labels under different names. If you see "natural flavorings", "hydrolyzed protein" and "spices" in a food label you are probably seeing a hidden way to "report" MSG in a food label, so be aware of the presence of MSG on foods that you thought were MSG free.

How Does MSG work

It has long been known that there are four basic tastes sweet, sour, salty, and bitter. It is now established that there is a fifth taste, called "Umami." Umami is the savory taste that occurs naturally in foods such as tomatoes and ripe cheese. Just as eating chocolate stimulates the sweet taste receptors on our tongue, eating food seasoned with MSG stimulates the glutamate or "umami" receptors on our tongue, enhancing the savory flavor of these foods.

MSG gives a "drug effect to the tongue," causing people to want to eat more. This is partly because of the taste and also because it triggers our brain causing the production of excessive amounts of dopamine. This creates a drug-like rush that provides a brief sensation of well being. It is highly addictive, causing its consumers to keep coming back for more and end up overeating. In the process, brain cells are destroyed. Because MSG damages the brain and therefore alters the ability of the brain to respond to the signal from the hormone leptin which in turn evokes an insatiable desire for more food and hence a prime culprit for obesity.

MSG also stimulates the pancreas to produce insulin into the blood stream even when there are not any carbohydrates in the blood for the insulin to act on. So insulin acts on the sugar present in the blood. Our blood sugar drops because of this flood of insulin, and then we end up hungry again an hour or so later. "No matter how much Chinese food we eat, we still end up hungry an hour later."

MSG : Its Effects

MSG functions not only as a flavor enhancer, but as a harmful neurotoxin or excitotoxin, which basically means, a chemical substance that excite your neurons (brain cells) and that may cause its death. Following are the diseases linked with MSG:

- Alzheimer's and Parkinson's Disease
- Seizures
- Brain Cell Damage
- Allergies
- Rashes
- Asthma attacks
- Brain Tumors
- Autism
- Attention Deficit Hyperactive Disorder in children
- Burning, Numbness or Tingling in or around your mouth,
- Cancer
- Chest pain
- Confusion
- Damage to unborn child
- Death due to an MSG reaction

- Diarrhea
- Eye inflammation
- Flushing
- Free radical damage to your blood vessels (this can lead to a heart attack or a stroke)
- Headaches (including migraine headaches)
- Heart disease
- Memory loss
- Nausea
- Pressure or tightness in the muscles on face
- Fertility problems (for both men and women)
- Rapid, fluttering heartbeats
- Shortness of breath
- Stuttering or speech problems
- Sweating
- Swelling of the brain (brain edema)
- Type 2 Diabetes
- Weakness
- Weight gain (the weight you gain from eating MSG is very difficult to loose)

MSG also triggers a broad set of symptoms called "**Chinese Restaurant Syndrome**" Chinese restaurant syndrome is a collection of symptoms that some people experience after eating Chinese food which contain MSG.

Symptoms of CRS"(Chinese Restaurant Syndrome)

- Chest pain

- Flushing

- Headache

- Numbness or burning in or around the mouth

- Sense of facial pressure or swelling

- Sweating

Those most vulnerable to the effects of MSG are the elderly, children, infants and the unborn. MSG is able to pass from mother to unborn child. The best way to avoid MSG is to eat fresh foods with no additives. You can find seasonings, soups and sauces free of MSG . If you are using a recipe that calls for MSG you can use fresh lemon as a substitute.

ASPARTAME

What is Aspartame?

Aspartame is a common, FDA approved, artificial sweetener used in many low-calorie food and beverages. Aspartame is also very sweet, and is said to taste about 200 times sweeter than sugar, which means little needs to be added to products; unless it is cooked or heated as it will lose its sweetness. It is made by mixing phenylalanine (an essential amino acid), and aspartic acid (a non essential amino acid). Some of the more common marketing names of aspartame are nutra sweet, sugar free etc.

Aspartame Uses

Aspartame's main use is as an artificial sweetener for low calorie foods and beverages. Due to its extremely sweet feature, very little is needed to sweeten the product it is being used in, therefore it has virtually no calories when added to food and drinks. Aspartame is also sold in individual packets so people can buy and use it in place of sugar in foods and beverages such as cereals, coffee and desserts. People who consume or use aspartame include those who wish to lose weight by lowering their caloric intake, and who are on special diabetic diets. Aspartame is also not only used in food and beverages, it has also been used to flavor children's medications or vitamins.

Aspartame History

Aspartame is, by far, the most dangerous substance on the market that is added to foods.

It was discovered by accident in 1965 when James Schlatter, a chemist of G.D. Searle Company, was testing an anti-ulcer drug. Aspartame was approved for dry goods in 1981 and for carbonated beverages in 1983. It was originally approved for dry goods on July 26, 1974, but objections filed by neuroscience researcher Dr John W. Olney and Consumer attorney James Turner in August 1974 as well as investigations of G.D. Searle's research practices caused the U.S. Food and Drug Administration (FDA) to put approval of aspartame on hold (December 5, 1974).

In 1985 Monsanto purchased G.D. Searle, the chemical company that held the patent to aspartame, the active ingredient in nutra sweet. Monsanto was apparently untroubled by aspartame's clouded past, including a 1980 FDA Board of Inquiry, comprised of three independent scientists, which confirmed that it "might induce brain tumors."

The FDA banned aspartame based on this finding, But Searle Chairman Donald Rumsfeld (currently the Secretary of Defense) vowed to get it approved.

On January 21, 1981, the day after Ronald Reagan's inauguration, Searle re-applied to the FDA for approval to use aspartame as food sweetener, and Reagan's new FDA commissioner, Arthur Hayes Hull Jr., appointed a 5-person Scientific Commission to review the board of inquiry's decision.

It soon became clear that the panel will support the ban by a 3-2 decision, but Hull then appointed a sixth member on the commission, and the votes became equal. He then personally broke the tie in aspartame's favor. Hull later left the FDA under allegations of impropriety, served briefly as Provost at New York Medical College, and then took a position with Burston-Marsteller, the chief public relations firm for both Monsanto and GD Searle.

Since then aspartame is found in all the sugar free sweet products.

Common Aspartame Side Effects

Some of the more common side effects that have been reported after consumption of aspartame are:

- Headache
- Dizziness
- Sudden, unexplainable mood swings
- Vomiting and Nausea
- Abdominal cramps
- Vision problems
- Diarrhea
- Memory loss
- Fatigue
- Rash or hives
- Sleep disturbances
- Changes in heart rate

The following chronic illnesses can be worsened or triggered by aspartame.

- Brain tumors
- Epilepsy
- Chronic fatigue syndrome
- Multiple sclerosis
- Epilepsy
- Parkinson's disease
- Alzheimer's
- Mental retardation
- Lymphoma
- Birth defects
- Fibromyalgia
- Diabetes

Now that we are aware what havoc these flavor enhancers and sweeteners can create in our lives. The name MSG can very well stand for MASS SUICIDAL GENERATION instead of Mono Sodium Glutamate.

CHAPTER -SEVEN

WHY DO WE GET A DISEASE
(Part-II)

Thoughts are things. Your body is in fact a very powerful electromagnetic transmitter and a receiver of energy. Every thought you have, puts a powerful impact on the cells of your body.

Positive high vibrational thoughts can purge your body diseases. Negative stressful low vibrational thoughts can 'confer' your body a series of diseases.

Let's try to understand how thoughts get converted into physical equivalents in the body.

Q. What happens, when you are angry?

Step 1: Brain detects the emotion of the thought as anger and sends the signal of anger to the pituitary gland (refer picture on the next page)

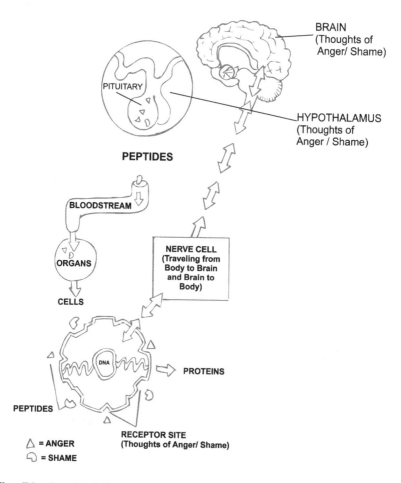

PITUITARY

PEPTIDES

BLOODSTREAM

ORGANS

CELLS

NERVE CELL
(Traveling from
Body to Brain
and Brain to
Body)

BRAIN
(Thoughts of
Anger/ Shame)

HYPOTHALAMUS
(Thoughts of
Anger / Shame)

DNA

PROTEINS

PEPTIDES

RECEPTOR SITE
(Thoughts of Anger/ Shame)

△ = ANGER
◠ = SHAME

The Biochemical Expression Of Anger / Shame And The Chemical /neurological Self Monitoring System Between The Brain And The Body.

Step II: Pituitary gland stimulates secretion of a kind of chemical (hormones) called Adrenaline (stress hormone) from the Adrenal glands, which through the blood stream reaches the different organs and gets attached to the cells of the different organs through receptor sites.

Step III: This results in the alteration of the functioning of the cells, leading to the physical changes in the outer body like sharpening of eyesight, and contraction of muscles in preparation of fight or flight. It also causes blood pressure and heart rate to increase, even as blood vessels constrict. When Adrenaline begins to flow through the body, digestion shuts down as blood is shunted away from the digestive tract and sent to the muscles.

When stress/anger is short-lived, a little burst of Adrenaline does more good than harm.

Step IV: In the long run repeated anger fits create a repeated imbalance in the energy management within the body, leading to a poor immunity. Many times extended stress or anger over a period results in a situation, where the body's defense mechanism is not able to distinguish between healthy cells and cancerous cells and starts killing all one by one, leading to a serious autoimmune diseases like Rheumatoid, Arthritis etc. It is a red carpet welcome for thousands of diseases.

I will make it simple for you. Imagine your home; assume there is some unpredicted call for emergency or threat in a part of the house. What will happen? As soon as the emergency call is heard, all the members of the house will rush towards that particular spot of the house, leaving the rest of the house, doors and windows unattended for a while, making the house vulnerable. At this moment it would be easier for a trespasser to enter and burgle the house or cause some or the other damage.

Your body is like your home and to attend calamity calls like stress, worry, tension, anger or any other negative emotion, it has to compromise with its inbuilt security system i.e. your body's immune system leading to the ingression of various diseases in the body.

'Remember, a positive attitude leads to a positive health.
Negative attitude leads, to a diseased body'.

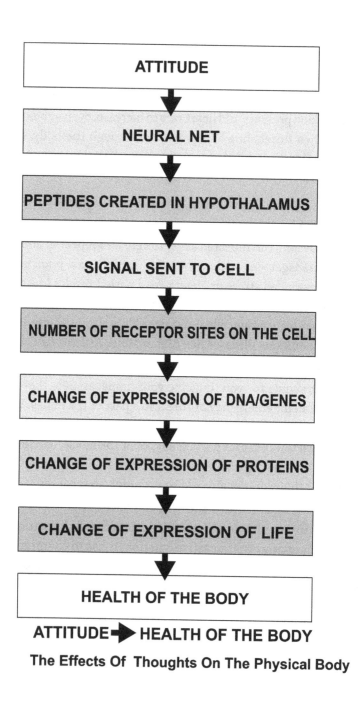

ATTITUDE

NEURAL NET

PEPTIDES CREATED IN HYPOTHALAMUS

SIGNAL SENT TO CELL

NUMBER OF RECEPTOR SITES ON THE CELL

CHANGE OF EXPRESSION OF DNA/GENES

CHANGE OF EXPRESSION OF PROTEINS

CHANGE OF EXPRESSION OF LIFE

HEALTH OF THE BODY

ATTITUDE ➡ HEALTH OF THE BODY

The Effects Of Thoughts On The Physical Body

CHAPTER -EIGHT

HOW NOT TO CURE A DISEASE!

Let's go back to the Mumbai Attack on the Taj Hotel where terrorists held the guests as the hostage and practically did every kind of damage to the beautiful building, guests, room occupants and the captive staff inside the Taj Hotel...

Most Insane Way to Solve the Problem:

What if poisonous gas is sprayed on the entire Taj Hotel. It would be filled with the poisonous gas. But for sure in this process the terrorists will die. What about captives and guests Oh Yes! they will also die in the process. Do you call it an intelligent way to combat with the crisis? No.. of course not......

This insane method was used by Russian Military on 23, Oct, 2002 when heavily armed Chechen Rebels held 129 person as a hostages, for 3 days in Moscow Theatre. Paralyzing gas was sprayed inside the theatre, resulting in the death of the 162 hostages as well as the rebels.

Only Way to Solve the Problem:

Intelligent solider who could identify and differentiate the terrorists from the guests should be sent inside the hotel. This will ensure the safety of the guest as well as the elimination of the terrorists.

Most of the lifeless drugs are insane like the poisonous gas. Most of the times, it is unable to distinguish between the diseased and healthy cells. Attack on the healthy cells as well as diseased cells leads to even more serious complications, which we call 'side effects' (like Pyar Ke side Effects ..Tablets Ke Side Effects). Chemo therapy, in case of cancer is the classic example of it.

Remember, drugs are always with side effects. Lifeless drugs cannot give life, but definitely make life 'less'.

To Understand the above Statement, Consider the Following Experiment

Take a pot and put four kilos of soil and manure in it. Also put one little tiny seed, and water it daily. At the end of a year you will have a big plant.

Well, take the plant out, shake off the soil from the roots and weigh the soil. Guess what! You still have 4 kg of soil. The only thing you added was some water. If you were to measure the water, you may have added about 2 kg of water.

Theoretically, the plant should weigh no more than 2 kg, if it retained 100 percent of the water. But the plant weighs twenty two kg. Wow! What happened? How did twenty two kg of mass and matter magically appear? It didn't eat the soil, the 4 kg of soil is still there, and there were only two kg of water added. How did that plant appear out of virtually nothing! This is a very important point; think about it again. The plant, like all living things, was virtually created out of "energy".

Energy is an "invisible matter".

Human beings are the same. If you take a little baby and you weigh every bit of food that goes in and then subtract all the excretions that come out through the urine, stool, and sweating through the skin, you would see that, whatever goes in, comes out of the body. If 4 kg of food and water are put in, guess what? 4 kg of stuff comes out, but the little baby grows from 6 kg to 68 kg.

But everything that goes inside the body, all the liquids and everything we eat comes out of the body. How does that happen? Well guess what? Science really can't give you an answer. The answer is that we get the energy from the food, Sunlight and air, and that's how matter is generated - it's the energy.

Drugs mask the symptoms rather than curing and eliminating of a disease. Your symptoms may be a running nose, ear-ache, sore throat, diarrhea, vomiting, excessive perspiration, acidity, fever, etc. These are the symptoms, not the root cause of your problem. These symptoms are personification of body's special mechanism to clean itself of toxins. In other words, your body is attempting to eliminate the trash from your body in a natural way.

This is an excellent thing, because your body is undergoing a self healing process. Drugs hamper this functioning. They not only arrest these symptoms, but also stop the cleansing process of the body. The toxins do not have means of expulsion, so they remain in the body.

If you run a high temperature, remember that your body is trying to kill the microbes (germs) inside you. It is exceptional that you need to bring down the fever (in a few cases it becomes necessary). For e.g. in your car red light blinking indicates that petrol is about to be exhausted. Flickering red light is a symptom. What would you do? Will you just disconnect the wiring showing red light? Will that solve the problem? No.........It will only appear outwardly, as if the problem is solved.

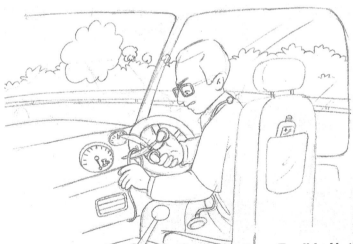

Disconnecting The Wire Signaling 'Low Fuel' Is Not A Solution Of The Problem.

Lifeless drugs just do the same.

Imagine an aquarium with healthy fishes dancing and moving fast from one corner to the other, but with the passage of time the water in the aquarium gets contaminated and the fishes start falling sick. What will you do?

Option 1: You take out the fishes, treat them and put them back in the aquarium.

Option 2: You replace the contaminated water with fresh water.

In so called modern hospitals and advanced medical science, you can expect the option 1.

Think about it. A person is suffering from a kidney failure..............

What will hospital's doctor do?

They will replace the defective, ailing kidney with the 'donor's kidney.

But in most of the cases it is discovered that within 3 to5 years, even the donor kidney gets infected, and becomes non-functional.

Until, we find the reasons of kidney failure, a permanent cure will never happen and cannot be achieved. We need to eliminate the root cause of the disease, not merely the symptoms.

So now we can say that a 'disease' is mainly an upshot of two factors-

1. When we eat a lifeless food.

2. When we have prolonged negative thoughts.

Unfortunately even the so called ultra modern hospitals do not treat any of the above causes.

Remember hospitals are not about health, but they are all about diseases.

To prove to yourself read through some of the authentic facts about the modern medicine system all over the world:

Fact 1: The main cause of death in the developed countries is not cancer or heart attack, but the side-effects of the drugs prescribed for curing diseases. It is called iatrogenic death.

In the USA, the number of deaths due to iatrogenic effect is more than the total deaths in wars since the commencement of the American history.

Fact 2: Statistically, medical doctors have an average life span of 65 years; where as the average life span of a common man is 75 to 80 years. Medical doctors are having the highest suicidal rate world wide. The average life span of a dentist is 52 years.

Fact 3: (a) Cancer victims going for chemo therapy and radiation have a survival rate of 3%.

(b) Cancer patient denying all kinds of treatment have a survival rate of 27%.

© Cancer patients going for alternative therapies have survival rate of 50%.

Mind boggling...Think over it.

Fact 4: The word 'Pharmacy' came from the Greek root word Pharmacia, which means sorcery or witchcraft. The word pharmacist means poisoner.

CHAPTER -NINE

SUMMARY TILL NOW

There are just two primary causes of a disease:

1) The negative/dead food.

2) The negative thoughts.

The healing in true sense is possible only, if the above two causes are eliminated from our life.

A so called hospital can truly be called a hospital, if it addresses the above two causes. Majorly the treatment only focuses on eliminating the symptoms not the causes.

Since only the symptoms are gone, but the cause is still there, once the effect of drug goes away, the symptoms appear again. But this time, you will need a bigger dose to subside the symptoms, since all drugs are addictive in nature.

Now the most imperative question of the life...

Q. To get ourselves completely healed and to remain healthy life long who should be turn to?

Answer: Just read on.

*"Science can repair something
which it has created
Science can not repair a thing which
it has not created."*

*"Nature has created us,
so the power to heal us
is within the nature itself."*

No one has the power to heal you, neither doctors, nor drugs have 'that power'. It is only within you and in the nature around you.

Important Fact: Herbivorous wild animals never die of serious diseases like heart attack, cancer, diabetes, migraine. Even if they fall sick, they get cured on their own, without the intervention of a doctor (except in case of accidents). These animals find a refuge in nature and cure themselves.

Have you ever seen a lion walking down the stairs of Escorts ...or a bunny going to an optician for a pair of glasses.

Considering all these examples, evidences and experiences, it's a time to take a pause...

And start building (or creating...) a true hospital, which can take care of both the factors responsible for causing any disease.

Factor 1:   Too much intake of negative food, results in the accumulation of many acidic toxins in the body and nutritional deficiency.

Factor 2:   Pent-up mental and emotional stress.

To build a "true" hospital only two associates can help you-

1. You yourself

2. Nature

You and nature together can build what may be called as the '***Super Specialty Home Hospital'.***

CHAPTER -TEN

THE SCIENCE OF SUPER HEALTH SIMPLIFIED

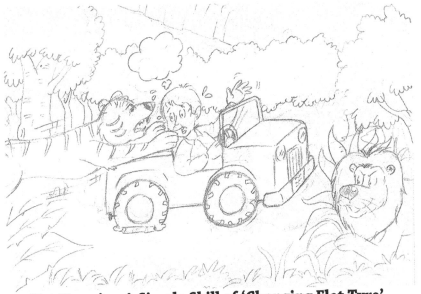

Not Knowing A Simple Skill of 'Changing Flat Tyre' Can Prove Perilous

Visualize that you are driving a car, crossing a huge forest, enjoying the unpolluted, clean weather & lush green scenic beauty. In the middle of the dense forest, suddenly you find that you have a flat tyre and you need to replace it fast, in order to avoid yourself to be placed on the 'menu card' of non- vegetarian animals.

Although changing a tyre is a very simple skill, neither you require a Phd degree in Automobile Engineering nor you need to be extra ordinarily enterprising and intelligent, but at this critical point of time not knowing this 'simple skill' can prove perilous and even fatal. You could be a delicacy of dinner for a tiger, lion or any carnivore ...

You may be killed, with no fault of yours. Your only slip or fault is that you never tried to learn the basic *first aid* of the car. So over dependence on the mechanic for minor car repairing can be taxing on your life...

Similarly you are a spirit living in the body. You must not be dependent at all on other persons to repair and maintain your body. After all it is a matter of life.

You must be thinking that do I mean that, we all must spend about a decade to learn about Human Body and Medicine? I don't mean that and actually it is not required also. God has created our body in a very systematic and simpler manner, we need only to understand it.

For example, we all human beings and most of the animals are comfortable living in a condition, where the temperature is between 15° C to 30° C (depends upon adaptability of an organism).

If it fluctuates by 20°C, body will be able to survive, but if the temperature is more than 100° C, the body will get burned and ultimately it will get destroyed. The organs and the cells of our body function in a similar manner.

As we understand for every object, there is a specific range of temperature at which it is in its best form. For example ice-creams are at their best at 15°C. The green tea tastes best at 79°-87° C. Similar to the temperature scale, for various fluid (like water, blood or urine) of the body, there is a different scale of measurement to understand the health status of the body. It is called the pH scale.

Definitions:

pH = measure of how much a substance is acidic or basic (alkaline)

pH scale = scale of measurement for acidity and alkalinity.

Understanding pH

pH (potential of hydrogen) is a measure of the acidity or alkalinity of a solution. It is measured on a scale of 0 to 14—the lower the pH, the more acidic the solution. The higher the pH, the more alkaline (or base) the solution. When a solution is neither acid nor alkaline it has a pH of 7 which is neutral.

Water is the most abundant compound in the human body, comprising 70% of the body. The body has an acid-alkaline (or acid-base) ratio called the pH, which is a balance between positively charged ions (acid-forming) and negatively charged ions (alkaline-forming.) The body continually strives to balance pH. When this balance is compromised many problems occur.

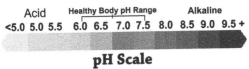

pH Scale

All chemical processes have an ideal pH at which they are the most efficient. For example the body functions at its best with an internal chemistry being slightly alkaline (pH of 7.0 to 8.0). The pH of the blood is even more specific:

Blood pH

pH 7.4 = Normal

Below 7 = May cause death

Our internal body chemistry functions in an alkaline environment. Our blood must maintain a pH of 7.4, if pH drops below 7 we may die.

The cells of a healthy body are alkaline. In disease, the cell pH is below 7.0. More acidic the cells become, sicker we are. The cells can survive pH above 3.5. pH below 3.5 it is fatal for cells.

Our bodies produce acids as a by-product of normal metabolism. Ironically body does not produce base, (for which the body strives) they must be supplied from outside to save cells from becoming acidic and dead.

Food is an important mean to stock up alkalinity in body. The main determining factor of alkalinity is the organic minerals. One can equate organic minerals with alkaline for better understanding. Foods are of two types, acid or alkaline. This refers to the ash value of a food. (Meaning the type of residue that remains after the food is digested and processed). Is it acid, or is it alkaline? If there is an acid residue (inorganic acids), the body must neutralize this acid to keep the blood from getting acidic. The acid is neutralized with alkaline.

Ideally, there is an adequate alkaline stuff in the diet to do this. However, if there is not, the body must extract alkaline from its cells to neutralize the acid. This tends to make cells acidic in due course and prone to illness.

As our bodies are basically an alkaline entity, in order to maintain good health, our diet must consist of alkaline ash foods.

The innumerable names of diseases do not really matter. What does matter is that they all come from the same root cause...too much Acid waste in the body.

Chart Of The Acidic And Alkaline Foods (Refer Page No. 44):

NOTE: Foods in the Acid Ash Column are listed in order of least acid to most acid; in the alkaline ash column, foods are listed in order from most alkaline to least alkaline.

Food Category	Most Alkaline	Alkaline	Lowest Alkaline	Lowest Acid	Acid	Most Acid
Sweeteners		Maple Syrup, Rice Syrup	Raw Honey, Raw Sugar	Processed Honey, Molasses	White Sugar, Brown Sugar	NutraSweet, Equal, Aspertine, Sweet 'N Low
Fruits	Lemons, Watermelon, Limes, Grapefruit, Mangoes, Papayas	Dates, Figs, Melons, Grapes, Papaya, Kiwi, Berries, Apples, Pears, Raisins	Oranges, Bananas, Cherries, Pineapple, Peaches, Avocados	Plums, Processed Fruit Juices	Sour Cherries	Blueberries, Prunes
Beans Vegetables Legumes	Asparagus, Onions, Vegetable Juices, Parsley, Raw Spinach, Broccoli, Garlic	Okra, Squash, Green Beans, Beets, Celery, Lettuce, Zucchini, Sweet Potato,	Carrots, Tomatoes, Fresh Corn, Mushrooms, Cabbage, Peas, Potato Skins, Olives, Soybeans, Tofu	Cooked Spinach, Kidney Beans, String Beans	Potatoes (without skins), Beans	Chocolate
Nuts Seeds		Almonds	Chestnuts	Pumpkin Seeds, Sunflower Seeds	Cashews	Peanuts, Walnuts
Oils	Olive Oil	Oil	Oil	Corn Oil		
Grains Cereals			Amaranth, Millet, Wild Rice,	Sprouted Wheat Bread, Spelt, Brown Rice	White Rice, Corn, Oats, Rye	Wheat, White Flour, Pastries, Pasta
Meats				Cold Water Fish	Turkey, Chicken, Lamb	Beef, Pork, Shellfish
Eggs Dairy		Breast Milk	Soy Cheese, Soy Milk, Goat Milk, Goat Cheese, Whey	Eggs, Butter, Yogurt, Buttermilk, Cottage Cheese	Raw Milk	Cheese, Homogenized Milk, Ice Cream
Beverages	Herb Teas,	Green Tea	Ginger Tea	Tea	Coffee	Beer

Chart Showing Alkaline and Acid Food

Testing the Salivary pH :

Optimal pH of saliva is above pH 7. If it is less than that it means the body is acidic and it's persistence for long, is a 'loving' invitation to illness. Just check the pH of early morning saliva, if it is above 7, means petering out of many ailments.

How to maintain salivary pH above 7:

1. Have 80% or more alkaline food and less than 20% acidic food (see chart)

2. 8 hours of restful sleep, during sleep many acid waste are processed and eliminated from the body through deeper breathing than we hardly ever allow ourselves in senses. Deep sleep is alkaline in nature.

3. At least ½ hr of any physical exercise is required to maintain an alkaline medium in the body.

4. Stress is always acid producing. Similarly any kind of negative emotion like fear, anger, hatred etc are all acidic in nature. STAY AWAY FROM THEM.

5. Love, peace, joy, calmness, forgiveness, something to believe in, a passion for life, and something within your life that is yours and yours alone, to feel passionate about are the ways to re-alkalize yourself.

6. Drink 8 to 10 glasses of water per day.

Special Note on Water:

One of the main causes of fatigue, toxemia (contamination of blood), constipation and premature aging is simply because most of the people don't drink enough water.

Water is involved in every metabolic process, electrical exchange and biochemical pathway, physical and mental activity of the body. It extracts nutrients from food, transports these nutrients to the blood, replenishes vital fluids, and helps to detoxify your body.

Three quarters of your body is composed of water. Your muscles are 70% water, blood is 82% to 90% water, bones are 35% water, liver is 90% water, and brain is 85% water.

If your body doesn't get enough water, it must recycle (reabsorb) what it already has by re-filtering it through the kidneys, putting an undue burden on the kidneys and the liver. It causes constipation too.

To understand the intensity of the above reasons, imagine that the supply of drinking water in your house, or say the whole city is disrupted for few days. Initially you will try to manage with the reserves you have, but once they are exhausted then! To survive one will try to filter the water remains of the drain and lastly the sewage system and the gutter to get the drinking water .... Extreme !I know you may say that you will prefer to die of dehydration than drinking water filtered from gutter.

That's the point. We must drink enough water so that our body never requires re-filtering of stored water from various organs of the body and in this way your kidneys and liver will be saved from the overtime.

Dehydration is one of the main cause of chronic pains such as headaches, arthritis, and a host of others. This is because of the concentration of acids and toxins re-circulating in the body, and also because of the drying of the lubricating layer of interfacial tissue, causing friction, which aggravates tissue inflammation and pain in many parts of the body.

Researches show that about 8-10 glasses of water per day may significantly ease back pain and joint pain up to 80% of sufferers.

If an average person drinks merely 5 glasses of plain water per day, the risk of getting breast cancer is decreased by as much as 79%, colon cancer by 45% and bladder cancer by 50% (water in your coffee, tea, sodas, etc. does not count towards daily water needs, as they are so acidic that they aggravate the problem, rather than solve it).

Soft drinks are extremely toxic. Studies have shown that heavy consumption of soft drinks (with or without sugar) spill out huge amounts of calcium, magnesium and other trace minerals from our body leading to osteoporosis, osteoarthritis, hypothyroidism, coronary artery disease, high blood pressure, premature aging and so on.

Moreover, it causes an abnormal acidic environment in our digestive system. The phosphoric acid present in soft-drink competes with hydrochloric acid of the stomach and affects its function badly. When the acid becomes ineffective, food remains undigested causing indigestion, gassiness and bloating.

Apart from this, it contains a common preservative known as Sodium Benzoate used in large quantity to prevent mould growth in soft-drinks and has the ability to switch off vital parts of DNA. ..A long list of diseases is tagged with a bottle of soft drink...so...it's not clear, no seedhi baat, still will you say Ye Dil Mange More...

CHAPTER -ELEVEN

SUPER SPECIALTY HOME HOSPITAL (THE SOLDIERS) STEP-1

To understand the steps of building 'Super Specialty Home Hospital' let's go back to the story of Mumbai attacks.

Imagine yourself to be the Taj Hotel once again, and the toxins as terrorists entering the beautiful Taj.

Let's jot down the problems to be combated:

1) Wiping out the terrorists and cleaning off the Taj Hotel.

2) Repairing the damages caused by the terrorists internally.

3) Safety of the hostages inside the hotel.

4) Ensuring the future safety of the hotel from the terrorist attack.

Solution: We need the following for the solution:

1) **Soldiers:** Intelligent and powerful soldiers, who can not only overpower and kill the terrorists, but are also able to identify and safeguard the hostages from the clutches of the terrorists.

2) **Repairmen:** Various damages like burnt parts of the hotel, smashed doors and windows, damaged electric lines (to cut the electric supply etc.) done by the terrorists. This means we need a range of repairmen with multifarious skills to repair, reconstruct and restore the original beauty of the Taj Hotel.

3) **Supreme Power**: Those terrorists were just the puppets controlled by

their commanders, sitting at a remote place. It is just the negative and polluted thought in which the terrorists were totally immersed up to such an extent that they were ready even to be killed for their mission. Here we need a supreme power, which can create a positive effect on terror community.

Q. Who can play the role of the soldier in our body, so that it can fight with the toxins and the poisonous matters inside the body and clean the body from the terrorists and also safe guard the healthy cells and organs from the injuries?

Ans. Look around yourself almost 1/3 of the Earth is covered with grass. Nature has given the 'soldiers' to animals and humans as cure in the form of grass. You might have seen cats and dogs nibbling over the grass whenever they fall sick. Intuitively animals know the grass is a cure for all kinds of sickness.

Among all types of grasses, wheat grass (till first 2 weeks after the germination of the wheat grains) has all the necessary nutrients capable of curing almost all kinds of diseases found on this Earth.

What is Wheat Grass?

Wheat grass refers to a product typically grown with wheat grain, in trays and juice extracted from wheat grass is consumed for healthy maintenance or treatment of any disease.

Wheat grass juice is a soldier in a true sense, a soldier equipped with all kinds of intelligence, power, sharpness and speed.

It can be called as a soldier of the body and has the greatest potential to cure the human body from practically every kind of disease, because of the following qualities:-

1) It is a complete protein containing over 20 essential and non- essential amino acids.

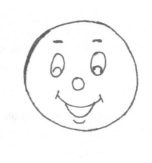

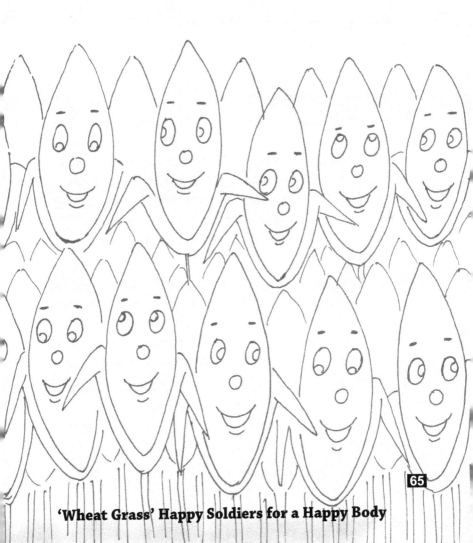

'Wheat Grass' Happy Soldiers for a Happy Body

2) In the Vitamin department, it contains twice Vitamin A (Beta-Carotene) than carrots, all the Vitamins B including B-12, more Vitamin C than oranges, Vitamin E and Vitamin K.

3) Wheatgrass is an excellent source for all major and minor minerals, containing 92 of the 102 minerals found in the soil. It is especially high in calcium, magnesium, manganese, phosphorus and potassium, as well as trace minerals such as zinc and selenium.

4) It contains essential fatty acids: Linolenic Acid and Linoleic Acid.

5) It has more than 80 different enzymes.

Nutritive value of 15 kg wheatgrass juice is equivalent to 350 kg of the choicest vegetables.

The Magic of Wheatgrass Juice

Wheatgrass has oxygen in diffusible state (ready for body absorption) in abundance. When we drink wheatgrass juice, supply of oxygen in blood increases, leading to the longevity and vitality of the body. Wheat grass contains raw chlorophyll. Chlorophyll is in fact, condensed sunlight. Since we are light beings having spirit and soul inside bodies, the light force vibrates through the physical body, that's the energy you feel. That's why wheatgrass is a spiritual food. It nourishes you on spiritual level as well as physical level.

Chlorophyll of wheatgrass is also known as green blood. When compared to the molecule of hemoglobin, the oxygen carrier in human blood, chlorophyll is almost identical. The major difference is that the nucleus of chlorophyll contains Magnesium (Mg), whereas hemoglobin contains Iron (Fe). (Refer chemical structure of blood and chlorophyll on next page)

Chlorophyll's unique ability to kill anaerobic odour producing bacteria is the reason, it covers up the smell of garlic, fights bad breath, body odor and acts as a general antiseptic. These bacteria, which live without air, are destroyed by chlorophyll's oxygen producing agents.

Chemical Structure of Blood & Chlorophyll

Dr. Otto Warburg, the 1931 Nobel Prize winner of Physiology and Medicine discovered that oxygen deprivation was a major cause of cancer. The cancer therapy today bombards tumours with ozone, a highly active oxygen. Unlike many drugs, chlorophyll has never been found to be toxic in any dosages.

Chlorophyll can even protect us from harmful radiation from X-ray, television, computer screen, transmitters and microwave. Famous research scientist E.Bircher called Chlorophyll as "Concentrated Sun Power" and reported that it increases the function of the heart, vascular system, kidneys, intestine, uterus and the lungs.

It raises the basic nitrogen exchange. And is therefore a tonic which, considering its stimulation properties cannot be compared with any other food or medicine on the planet. We can conclusively say that drinking wheatgrass juice certainly detoxyfies the blood and strengthens the immune system. It leads to more energy and an improved ability to combat and reverse illness.

Some of the Nutrients in Wheat Grass

Amino Acids:

Typtophan, Glutamic Acid, Alanine, Methionine, Arginine, Lysine, Aspartic Acid, Cystine, Glycine, Hisidine, Isoleucine, Leucine, phenylalaine, Proline, Serine, Threonline, Valine.

Enzymes:

(Over 80 have been identified) Super-oxide Dismutase, Peroxidase, Phosphatase, Catalase, Cytochrome Oxidase, DNase, RnaseSuperoxide, Hexokinase, Malic dehydrogenase, Nitrate reductase, Nitrogen oxyreductase, Fatty Acid Oxyreductase, Fatty Acid Oxidase, Phosolipase, Polyphenoloxidase, Dismutase, Transhydrogenase.

Phytochemicals: Chlorophyll, Carotenoids, Bioflavonoids, growth hormones, RNA, DNA.

Vitamins:

Vitamin C, Vitamin E (Succinate), Beta-carotene (Vitamin A) Biotin, Choline, Folic Acid, B1-Thiamine, B2-Riboflavin, B3-Niacin, B6-Pantothenic Acid and Vitamin K.

Minerals & Trace Minerals:

Zinc, Selenium, Phosphorus, Potassium, Calcium, Boron, Chloride, Chromium, Cobalt, Copper, Iodine, Iron, Magnesium, Nickel, Sodium and Sulfur.
(These are the primary ones, there are many more.)

Fatty Acids:

Linolenic Acid, Linoleic Acid.

Per 100 grams		Grass	Sprouts	Broccoli	Eggs	Chicken
Protein	g	25	7.490	2.980	12.440	17.550
Fat	g	7.980	1.270	.350	9.980	20.330
Calcium	mg	321.000	28.000	48.000	49.000	10.000
Iron	mg	24.9000	2.140	.880	1.440	1.040
Magnesium	mg	112.000	82.000	25.000	10.000	20.000
Phosphorus	mg	575.000	200.000	66.000	177.000	172.000
Potassium	mg	3,225.000	169.000	325.000	120.000	204.000
Sodium	mg	18.800	16.000	27.000	280.000	71.000
Zinc	mg	4.870	1.650	.400	1.100	1.190
Copper	mg	0.375	.261	.045	.014	.074
Manganese	mg	2.450	1.858	.229	.026	.019
Selenium	mg	2.500	n/a	3.000	30.800	n/a
Vitamin	mg	214.500	2.600	93.200	0.000	2.400
Thiamin	mg	0.350	.225	.065	.049	.114
Riboflavin	mg	16.900	.155	.119	.430	.167
Niacin	mg	8.350	3.087	.638	.062	6.262
Pantothenic	mg	0.750	.947	.535	1.125	.920
Vitamin B	mcg	1.400	.265	.159	.118	.330
Folate	mcg	1,110.000	38.000	71.000	35.000	6.000
Vit. B-12	mcg	0.800	0.000	0.000	.800	.320
Vitamin A	IU	513.000	0.000	n/a	632.000	178.000
Vit A, RE	mcg	2,520.000	0.000	154.000	190.000	52.000
Vitamin E	mg	9100	.050	1.660	1.050	n/a

Vitamin & Mineral Comparison of Wheat Grass & Common Foods

Some Benefits of Grass Substantiated By Research

> Repairs DNA	> Reduces Cholesterol
> Enhances Immunity	> Prevents Inflammation
> Stops Free-Radicals	> Promotes Cellular Rejuvenation
> Inhibits Carcinogens	> Enhances Stamina & Endurance
> Increases Longevity	> Neutralizes Pesticides
> Provides Growth Hormone	> Provides Antioxidants
> Helps to Cure Skin Diseases	> Lowers Atherosclerosis Risk

The blade of grass contains all the revitalizing and rebuilding materials of which the body is composed of. It is a producer of energy and eliminator of waste acids. Grass is the perfect food.

Grasses are a complete life sustaining food. Based on the animal studies, if you had to choose one food for survival, it ought to be only wheat grass. After all, grasses are the primary food for domestic and wild grazing animals and even for some pretty large ones like elephants, rhinoceros and hippopotamus etc.

Frequently Asked Questions:

Question: How do I avoid mould when growing wheatgrass?

Answer: Mould is the most common problem, when growing wheatgrass (in fact it is often the only problem). It can be identified as white blobs forming (normally around the base of the wheatgrass stalks) when it is alive and as black spots when it is dead. The following are the suggestions for preventing mould formation to your home grown wheatgrass.

1) Do not soak your wheatgrass grains for longer than 12 hours (extreme cold conditition is an exception where you may have to soak the wheat grains for even more than 24 hrs).

2) Do not keep the sprout bag in water bowl, it will initiate mould formation.

Question: At what stage the wheat grass should be used for Juice?

Answer: The plant undergoes rapid growth with increasingly nutritional manifestation until maturity (when it switches gear from vegetative growth to reproductive growth). Just prior to this change- over, the plant is at its nutritional peak. This transition is known as jointing (as shown in picture). After jointing the nutritional counts drop radically. The plant then start sending all its nourishment to the developing wheat grains.

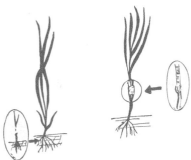

Think of jointing as a kind of puberty for plant. At this stage it has maximum nutritional value

Question: Can I take wheatgrass during my pregnancy?

Answer: Wheatgrass is great for prenatal care, as it provides the body with nutrients like antioxidants, chlorophyll and folic acid.

Question: I have a wheat or gluten allergy, is wheatgrass juice safe to take?

Answer: Wheatgrass is harvested till the jointing stage, before it turns into a grain. In this stage the grass does not contain any gluten. It is extremely rare for people with wheat allergies to have reaction, because they are usually allergic to the gluten found in the wheat kernel. Wheat grain is different than wheat grass. One is grain and other is a green vegetable.

Question: Can you use wheat grass powder instead of Wheat grass Juice?

Answer: The Wheat grass juice has all the nutrients capable to fight with diseases found in our body, more over it is also mandatory to consume the juice within twenty minutes of the preparation. After that time period the nutrient value radically falls down, but in case of wheat grass powder, the optimum benefit can not be attained. Anything that is dried has an incredible loss of vital life force. Even if you dry it carefully. Dried is dormant. Dormant is inactive. Problem with all that dried stuff is the life force. The ethereal energy is dissipated and lost. You are something highly vibrational and wheat grass juice is also the highly vibrational –it tunes right into you and brings up your vibration.

Question: How can I take out the wheat grass juice?

Answer: The best way to extract juice is to use special kind of juicer particularly meant for wheat grass only. Other way is to use a mortar and pestle for taking out juice. For more information you can contact at the following address:

India Book of Records,
B-121, 2nd Floor, Green Field,
Faridabad-121003,
Ph.:+91-129-2510534,
E-mail:indiabookofrecords@gmail.com,
www.indiabookofrecords.in

CHAPTER -TWENTY

SUPER SPECIALTY HOME HOSPITAL (THE REPAIRMAN) STEP -2

Once the Taj Hotel is freed from the terrorists, now it needs to be revamped, renovated and darned..... Now it needs repair .....

Humans, metaphorically 'The Taj', too need revamping and restoration for good health. For human body the following panacea can play the role of 'repairmen' to restore and repair the damage, due to constant intake of poor and negative food and unhealthy thought processes over the years.

1. **Tulsi : Some Facts about Tulsi:**

   - Protects from nearly all sorts of infections from viruses, bacterias, fungi and protozoas.

   - An excellent anti biotic, fungicidal, germicidal, disinfectant, very efficiently protects the body.

   - Leaves extract keep mosquitoes and other insects away.

   - Contains vitamin C and other anti oxidants (such as Eugenol), which protect the heart from harmful effects of free radicals.

   - Soothes nerves, lowers blood pressure, reduces inflammation and thus reduce stress.
   - It is very beneficial in reducing cholesterol from blood.
   - Effective in curing nearly all types of respiratory disorders including bronchitis (chronic and acute).
   - Beneficial in asthma, and relieves congestion and facilitates breathing.
   - Cures congestion of the lungs.
   - Destroys most of the germs and bacteria in the mouth and this effects last long.

'Rock n Roll' with Honey, Amla, Garlic, Ginger, Lemon and Tulsi

74

2. **Garlic: Some Facts about Garlic**
   - Eases constricted breathing in asthma.
   - Reduces frequency or severity of convulsions.
   - Fights infection, especially in the digestive and respiratory tracts.
   - Combats cramping and spasmodic pains, especially in the digestive tract.
   - Kills intestinal worms.
   - Stimulates sexual desire.
   - Helps expel gas.
   - Promotes sweating and circulation to the skin.
   - Stimulates digestion.
   - Directly kills germs.
   - Promotes urination.
   - Balances menstruation.
   - Promotes the flow of mucous, improving the productivity of coughs.
   - Irritating to the skin, and thus will draw blood supply to an area of the body, when applied over that area.
   - Increases short-term energy.
   - Improves overall health and strength, when taken regularly.

3. **Lemon: Some Facts about Lemon**
   - Rich in citric acid and vitamin C.
   - Repels free radicals and protects healthy cells from becoming cancerous, and is especially beneficial for smokers.
   - Promotes constant regeneration of bone tissue.
   - Stimulates the absorption of calcium and helps in the development of strong and healthy teeth.
   - Has small amount of iron and vitamin B-complex.
   - Has alkaline pH, so it helps in digestion of food.

4. **Honey: Some Facts about Honey**
   - Iron, copper, manganese, silica, chlorine, calcium, potassium,

sodium, phosphorus, aluminum and magnesium, all are present in honey.

- Contains minerals to balance the body.
- Contains predigested sugar which helps a person with a weak digestive system.
- Packed with the nutrients vital for body rejuvenation.
- Furnishes minerals which supplement those found in milk, as well as a small amount of protein.
- Maintains the blood sugar level.
- Prevents the raising of the blood pressure level in the body.
- High calorie content, can build up energy with small servings.
- Glucose in honey restores the oxygen that is replaced by lactic acid when fatigue sets in.
- Helps the body in building up tissues.
- Presence of Dextrin (type of sugar) in honey makes it easy to digest.

5. Ginger : Some Facts about Ginger

- Blocks the effects of prostaglandin – a substance that causes inflammation of the blood vessels in the brain and can lead to migraine.
- Effective for relieving the severity of nausea even in cases of pregnancy.
- Ginger helps to cure menstrual cramps.
- Anti-inflammatory properties that can lessen the pain of rheumatoid arthritis.
- Well known for its warming action on the upper respiratory tract
- Effective in cramps caused by stomach gas.
- Makes the platelets less sticky and is of great benefit in case of circulatory disorders.
- Acts as mood enhancer.
- Its Cineole acts as a stress relief.

6. Amla: Some facts about Amla

- It is a strong rejuvenative.
- It balances stomach acids.
- It improves food absorption.
- It is an anti-oxidant prevents premature aging.
- It prevents and treat respiratory disorders.
- It makes lungs strong and healthy.
- It enhances brain functions.
- It detoxifies and cleanses.
- It enhances fertility.
- It strengthens immune system.
- It acts as a coolant.
- It treats hemorrhage, diarrhea and dysentery.
- It is an anti-oxidant and has detoxification properties, amla is well known for treating skin disorders.
- It removes disorders of the eye.
- It prevents premature graying and falling of hair.

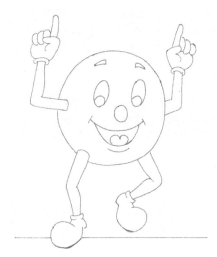

"Happy -go-Lucky' Life with Amla

7. Aloe Vera: Some facts about Aloe Vera

- Aloe vera is used to make facial moisturizers
- It is used to make hair gel.
- It helps in healing minor cuts and scrapes.
- It removes stretch marks from pregnancy and surgery.
- It helps in regenerating new skin cells.
- It is used to make dandruff removing cream.
- It helps in removing blackness under eye and wrinkles.
- It is used to heal rashes, burns, sores, blisters, acne, pimples, insect bites and sun burn.
- It is helpful in healing vaginal infections.
- It is helpful in healing fungus.
- It is helpful in healing conjunctivitis.
- It is helpful in healing allergic reactions.
- It is applied on dry skins to give them glowing effect.
- It is used to reduce psoriasis.
- It is used to reduce warts.
- It is used to reduce eczema.

Note: Aloin, also known as Barbaloin, it is a yellow-brown colored substance that is bitter to taste. It is found in the outer leaf of aloe vera plant. In 2002 the outer leaf, that contains Aloin, was banned by the Government of USA. It is always better to avoid Aloin in juices or consult a physician before starting to use aloin along with Aloe Vera . In rare cases, it may cause an allergic reaction, although Aloin is used to treat constipation, because it induces peristaltic contractions in the colon and leads to bowel movement, but it should be used under physician supervision.

CHAPTER -THIRTEEN

SUPER SPECIALTY HOME HOSPITAL (THE SUPREME POWER)STEP- 3

Years ago, NASA designed a fascinating experiment to test the physiological and psychological impact of special disorientation, the kind that astronauts might experience during extended time in a weightless environment. NASA outfitted a group of astronaut candidates with convex goggles that flipped everything in their field of vision by 180 degrees, so that the world they saw was completely upside down. The test subjects wore these glasses twenty four hours a day, even while asleep. Then the scientists sat back to observe what happened.

At first, extreme stress and anxiety were obvious as reflected in the astronaut's blood pressure along with other vital signs. The astronauts gradually adapted to this new level of stress, but it still didn't dissipate altogether. After all their entire world was upside down. But twenty six days after the experiment began, something amazing happened to one astronaut. His world turned upright again. The goggles hadn't changed and he was still wearing them continuously, but now he was able to see everything around him as normal. Within the next several days, all the other astronauts followed suit.

What had happened? After twenty one to thirty days of this constant stream of strange new inputs, men's brain had created enough new neural connections to completely rewire their brains, so that their visual and spatial perception worked at 180 degrees opposite from the way the brain normally works.

In repeated trails, the researchers also discovered that if the goggles were removed during this three to four week period, even for short times, the neural adaptation would not occur. In other words, it took about twenty five to thirty days of uninterrupted, consistent input of new perceptual (conscious) information for the subconscious brain to accept that it had to adjust to this new information and regard it as normal.

Our conclusion...! It takes about 21 to 30 days of consistently applying mental rehearsal for your subconscious brain to absorb a new orientation and our experience with thousands of clients over the past twenty years confirms this.

Mental Rehearsal System

Imagine you decide to run a marathon. You practically run or not, is a different question but when this idea strucked you, you knew that it needs lot of efforts and inputs. Running a marathon is not a cake walk that you decide one morning and by weekend you are all set for it.

It takes time, consistent, methodical efforts and of course equal amount of hard work and determination. You need to work out daily, breaking in your system bit by bit, toning and strengthening your muscles, training your lungs and heart, gradually acclimatizing your entire system to new habits of activity.

This is exactly what you're going to do with your brain. We are going to show you how to recondition and tone the neural networks in your brain so that they establish new habits that match up with new beliefs, so that your success happens naturally and organically from the inside out. We have developed a process called the Mental Rehearsal System that will help you take those goals and dreams and turn them into neural patterns in your subconscious brain, as opposed to simply writing them down for your conscious brain and then forgetting about them.

Just like when you are getting ready to run a marathon, this process will condition and tone your neural system to do what it takes to achieve your dream business. And just like getting ready to run a marathon, this conditioning process is something that takes consistent daily effort. It is not a huge task, in fact it is almost ridiculously easy to do. It's just that most people don't do it. But you will and that will make all the difference.

5 STEPS OF MENTAL REHEARSAL SYSTEM
Step One: Create A New Vision

Your subconscious brain retains the memory of everything you have ever witnessed or experienced; what's more, it retains the memory of everything you have ever imagined. Remember, your subconscious brain does not distinguish between experiences that are "real" and events that happened only in your mind. When you imagine a vivid experience, in neurological terms it has taken place, and your brain views its every bit as real as your hand or the chair you're sitting on.

It was only natural that I would end up breaking a world record in push - ups by doing 198 push ups in a minute, because as far as my subconscious brain was concerned, after imagining that I am doing 200 push - ups a minute thousand of times, the belief system of my brain saw this as my real performance and it made sure my senses and conscious mind picked up on whatever actions it would take to put me there physically.

While your subconscious brain does not distinguish between extremely real or imagined event, what it does distinguish is how strongly it is imprinted. Memories that have carved a deeper channel in your brain, regardless of whether they are actual or imagined events, have a great influence than those of lesser imprint.

What determines the strength an imprint? The same two factors that dictate the power of any memory: repetition and impact – are emotional content. Both factors are crucial.

Repetition

Repetition is simple: You don't create a habit by doing something once. You create a habit by doing that something over and over. This is how you learned to walk, to talk and to do your multiplication tables. Repetition creates habit and this is also true for your habits of thought.

This is one major reason why people so often fail to achieve the goals they set. You can sit in a seminar and declare a goal, take pen and paper on January 1 and write down a New Year's resolution but doing that once means next to nothing. The only way it stands the slightest chance of coming true is if it becomes a habit of thought – and the only way that stands the slightest chance of happening is if you repeat it, over and over, dozens of times. This is why the real power of mental rehearsal lays not so much in exactly how you do it; but that you do it every day, day after day, for weeks and so on ...

Impact

Repetition will create habit, even if there is no great emotion involved, but without the factor of emotional impact, the habit may be fairly shallow and not have much staying power. The reason for this is that there is a strong interaction between emotion and memory. Events that occur with a powerful emotional charge attached – say a time of great elation such as the birth of a child, or a traumatic car accident – have far more impact in the brain than the unexceptional lunch you had six months ago.

REPETITION + IMPACT = NEW REALITY

Let's say your goal is to win a gold medal at the Olympics. Here's what you do: Create a vivid picture in your imagination of what that experience would be. Like the feeling of standing up there on the podium with your national anthem playing, the crowd roaring with enthusiasm, the feeling of the blood pumping in your veins, the thrill and rush as Olympic official reaches up and hangs the medal around your neck. Can you feel it?

When you imagine all that in such vivid detail, you are evoking that experience and exposing it to your subconscious mind just as effectively as if you were actually standing on that podium with the whole world watching and that medal hanging around your neck.

Repeat this vividly and consistently enough and pretty soon you aren't just imagining you are an Olympic gold medalist but at a very real, visceral level, you are becoming a gold medalist. And because you are, you'll start doing what a gold medalist does, taking the actions a gold medalist takes, living the way a gold medalist lives, and attracting those circumstances that a gold medalist attracts.

If this at all sounds esoteric, all you have to do is ask any Olympic gold medalist if he ever spent any time visualizing himself taking that top medal. You better believe they have – every single one of them, over and over, every day, for years. It's a recipe for outstanding achievement that every top athlete, every award-winning musician, actor, or dancer, every famous speaker, president, CEO, or super successful businessperson knows.

When you visualize something, you are literally creating a pattern of neural network within your brain that corresponds to what it is you want to achieve. You are creating the seed that is required to start attracting those resonant resources necessary to allow that blueprint to unfold into its physical manifestation.

It's as simple as this: No seed, no tree. You want a tree? Visualization is how you create the right seed.

Step Two: Create Powerful Affirmations

Now that you have your crystal clear vision in place, you need to ensure that your daily routine even the jiffy beliefs are in line with what you say and you want to achieve. This step is critical... Why! Because if you try to realize a new vision, while maintaining old beliefs that do not support that vision, you've got a classic case of mixed messages.

For example, when a mother says "Come here, I love you," but her arms are folded and there is clearly anger or irritation in her voice, which message does the child receive! (Hint: It's not the words) That's right: When your words don't match your actions, feelings, moods, beliefs; the nonverbal will win out, every time.

This is exactly how it is with the conscious (verbal) and subconscious (nonverbal) brain: When the message your conscious brain puts out such as your written goals, competes with a message your sub-conscious brain holds to be true (your beliefs, even if they are unstated), guess which one will win out! You already know the answer.

In other words you may say, "I want to quadruple my business, from ₹250,000 per year to a million a year," but if your subconscious mind is still set on a quarter million dollar picture, then it's like saying "I love you," with your arms crossed and a scowl on your face. Again, whenever there's conflict between conscious and subconscious, the subconscious will always win.

So let's take a closer look at your underlying beliefs.

How do you know what your present beliefs are? This can be a tricky thing because our beliefs tend to be so much a part of us that we often aren't even aware of them. There is a wonderful ancient Hindu expression: "There are three mysteries in the world: the air to the bird, the water to the fish and man to himself." Fishes aren't aware of water: It's where they swim in all the time, so they don't think about it. Same with birds and air: It's their normal environment. And that's how our beliefs are: We swim in them all the time, so much so that they are typically invisible to us.

So how do you know what your beliefs are? The answer turns out to be incredibly simple: Just look at your life. What do you see? Whatever you find there's the evidence of your beliefs, your current life your relationships, your health, your income, your lifestyle, where you live, where you work, where you play, what you do every day, all of it- is an accurate reading of the picture you've been holding in your subconscious brain.

If you are broken, then your belief is, "I' m broken. I am a failure ...that's how I am made of, I can never be a successful man." Or, "I don't deserve to have lot of money."

If you are stressed out, pressured, never have enough time, then welcome this belief, "There is never enough time, I have to manage within this stipulated time and do all I can ."

Also do it...

If you feel like your life is satisfactory overall, but there's never quite enough time to do what you really want to do and never enough money to do what you want to do, then guess what belief are you holding?

"There is never quite enough." And if you are thinking, "Well, no, not right now, but definitely soon, eventually, someday." Then dear friends... I have a bad news for you: It will never happen... Reason! For your subconscious, there is no past and future, no after some time, no planning for future...but only the present moment, right now! If not now then your sub conscious brain will be forever trapped in "Someday" like a fly in amber.

The first step is to accept the fact that you are in the driver's seat: Your life is your creation, and the principal tool you have used to create it is your beliefs. If you want to change things and then decide what belief you want to have.

Creating Your Affirmations

The key to writing effective affirmations is that they must be bold, clear, positive and stated in the present tense.

We've explored the problem posed by the fact that people often articulate their goals in negative terms.

In other words, rather than focusing on what they want, they focus on what they don't want? "I want to be in a fulfilling lifelong relationship" and "I really don't want to end up sad and alone" might seem like two ways of saying the same thing. They're not. To your subconscious brain, they are contradictory. Your subconscious doesn't know the difference between "I want" and "I don't want." It just hears "lifelong fulfilling relationship" or "sad and lonely."

Your conscious brain puts things in logical, linear sequences. It has to, it can't focus on more than one or two things at a time. But your subconscious can focus on a million things at once. It doesn't need to think, "First this, then that, then eventually..." while your conscious brain might read a story from beginning to end, your subconscious brain just sucks up the entire story as one impression, You can see this with kids, especially young kids, who have had less time to develop sophisticated filters and defenses and often reveal the truth of their thought process far more innocently and openly than adults or older kids do. If you tell a child not to do something, what he will be drawn to do? Exactly what you told him not to do.

Let's say you want your child to get through a meal without spilling his milk. If you say, "Hey, make sure you don't spill your milk," have you decreased the chances that milk is going to spill? No, in fact, chances are good you've actually increased them.

The same is true for the things we say to ourselves, in fact it is hundreds of times more true. Why? Because you might tell your child not to spill his milk at most, what, once or twice a day? Three times?

But if you're giving yourself a similar warning- "whatever you do, don't get nervous" – how often will you repeat that to yourself in a single day? Easily hundreds of times. The things we say to ourselves, we say over and over, dozens, hundreds, thousands, tens of thousands of times. The one person you have by far the most influence over is you- because nobody whispers in your ear even a tiny fraction of the amount that you do yourself.

STEP THREE: CREATE EMOTIONAL ANCHORS FOR NEURAL LINKING

There is a technique called neural linking that uses the emotional association to deepen the impact of belief or affirmation you choose. You accomplish this by linking that new belief with powerful feelings that already exists in association with some other memory.

Neural linking happens to us all the time. How often have you come across a certain smell – the first cut grass in springtime, the burning leaves in autumn, a wool sweater pulled out of a closet, a certain dish on the stove that you haven't eaten in ages – and suddenly a full-fledged memory from the distant past came flooding back to you! This happens because memory is strongly associative by nature.

You can put that associative trait to work for you by designing specific links for yourself. Here's how you do that. First, search your memory bank for a positive event in your life that was especially empowering, a moment where you felt a thrill of accomplishment, excitement, or triumph. What you are looking for is an existing neural pattern in your brain that has some "stickiness," that is some strong depth of feeling to which a thought can adhere.

Jot down a sentence or two that identifies this event, so you can return to it easily and quickly later on.

Now, close your eyes and let yourself re-experience that event for a few moments and examine what you're seeing, hearing, smelling, feeling and experiencing.

When you're finished, jot down a few of the impressions you had; these don't need to be full sentences, just words or phrases that will remind you of the feelings this experience evokes; Now, choose one of your affirmations. Choose a statement that is fairly short and that you strongly want to imprint as a new belief. In my case, I chose, my strong muscles are able to complete 200 push-ups in a minute. Since this is definitely not a belief I grew up with and yet it has been critical to my achieving success in my business visions.

Now, close your eyes again and let yourself re-experience that powerful memory, evoking all the sensory impressions, feelings and emotions involved, and while you are at the height of that feeling, repeat your new affirmation, either out loud or just in your mind.

Here's what happens. When an event (whether "real" or in your mind) evokes strong emotions, a protein is released along with neurotransmitters. As the neurons fire across the synaptic gap and that cause the event to bind to that neural pathway much more strongly than if it was simply a neutral thought or memory. When you relive that powerful event and bring back that old feeling, you are physically bonding that new affirmations to that event into this existing neural pathway.

I'll share an example that I use for myself. It was July 21, 1999, the launch of my first book 'Dynamic Memory Methods' with Chief Justice of India, Justice M.N.Venkatachelliah as a chief guest. The hall was jam-packed with national electronic and print media and the people from literary world. I could still vividily remember the exhilarating rush of emotion, as I was signing the first autograph of my life to the first buyer of my book, who was none other than Ex- CBI Director Mr. Kartiken. It was one of the most emotional moments of my life, a feeling of being totally in the flow.

This feeling is so powerful, so vivid that I can go back there and re-experience that feeling and then I can think, "My strong muscles are able to complete 198 push-ups in a minute.

I attach that exhilarated feeling to this new belief that I want to instill, using the emotion and the neural pathways that are already in place, thereby associating that thirteen year old feeling, that is still so resonant in my mind, with this new belief.

STEP FOUR: PREPARE YOUR NEURAL IMPRINTING MATERIAL

Imprinting materials are simply physical expressions of your vision and affirmations that you can feed into your subconscious brain through your senses. The most common examples of imprinting material are:

- Written statements, typed and laminated
- Audio recordings, including simple voice recordings, voice over music recordings
- Pictures and vision boards

The whole process of designing your vision and affirmations of sitting down and writing them out, editing them, typing a clean copy, getting it laminated... all that preparation are your conscious brain's abilities. Now you get to use these tools to imprint these images onto your subconscious.

You can accomplish this routine in as little as thirty minutes a day. The more time you give to it, the more quickly your new vision and supporting beliefs will become ingrained at the subconscious level and the more quickly your goal will take the shape in the physical world of events and circumstances. Again, the most important thing is not how long you do it, but that you do it.

It's best to do this at roughly the same time every day, because your body is sensitive to its own circadian rhythms. This is a key to successful conditioning that every professional athlete, musician, dancer and writer knows. A routine practiced five days in a row at the same time every day has far greater impact on developing your abilities than a routine practiced five days in a row at widely different times.

The ideal time for this practice is when you are a little tired and not too focused. That half-awake/half-asleep state, when you don't have your conscious filters fully in place, is the moment when your subconscious is most accessible. Ideal timings are first thing upon rising in the morning, and last thing before going to sleep at night. We also recommend adding a third time during the day. This might be during your lunch break or whenever you can break off from the action of the day to find a few minutes of quiet seclusion. If you're someone who steals a few minutes midday to catnap, then that's the perfect time to add in your midday neural reconditioning.

It's also a good idea to practice this routine in the same place every day, if you can. Find a quiet and solitary place where you can be undisturbed for at least ten minutes. Turn off your phone, pager, email alert or anything else that might interrupt you.

STEP FIVE: FEEL THE DOUBT AND DO IT ANYWAY

As you first start going through this daily process, you may feel a nagging sense of discomfort, anxiety, or doubt. When you say "I am breaking a world record for.........................Category".

You may hear another voice in your head that says, "No you're not! Why are you lying!"

Don't let this throw you. This is completely normal. What you're feeling at this time is your psycho-cybernetic system doing what it's designed to do: alerting you to the fact that you're making a change in course. It's simply the 'lookout' in your brain, watching where you're headed and sending you an alert message: "Captain new goals, dead ahead! We're having five-hundred-thousand-dollar thoughts! We've changed course what should we do?"

The key is to feel it, sense it and appreciate the fact that your psycho-cybernetic system is doing its job, doing what it does to keep you safe – but don't interpret that with a "retreat!" response. Interpret it as the thrill of moving into new territory. Reply to your own message; I know, It's okay, that's exactly where we want to be headed. Full speed ahead! Let that sense of anxiety or discomfort translates into the thrill of adventure.

Final Dose of Inspiration

The easiest thing in the world is to find reasons or excuses of not achieving your goal. You could simply think that may be I am not as lucky or lacking proper finances and opportunity to train myself to achieve excellence. Remember our brain is like a search engine, whatever question we feed we get an answer. So try to feed positive questions. We are limited not by resources, but only by thoughts.

World's Fastest Man with no Feet

Oscar Leonard Carl Pistorius (born on 22 November 1986) is a South African Paralympic runner. Known as the "Blade Runner" and "the fastest man with no legs" who has a double amputation, is the world record holder in the 100, 200 and 400 metres (sport class T44) events and runs with the aid of Cheetah Flex-Foot carbon fibre transtibial artificial limbs by Ossur. In 2007 Pistorius took part in his first international competition for able-bodied athletes. At the 2008 Summer Paralympics, he took the gold medals in the 100, 200 and 400 metres (T44) sprints.

First Amputee Ever to Qualify for Olympics

Natalie du Toit (born on January 29, 1984) is a South African swimmer. She lost her leg in a motorbike accident. She is one of the world's most well-known para-athletes and has dominated disabled Swimming Championship in the last three Commonwealth Games and Paralympics. She was awarded 50m and 100m Freestyle Commonwealth title for elite athletes with a disability held in Manchester in 2002. Moreover she has 11 Paralympic gold medals and competed against able-bodied athletes in the 2008 Summer Olympics in Beijing. She has made history by becoming the first amputee to qualify for the Olympic Games, an achievement that defies scientific logic. She became the first disabled swimmer to compete in an able-bodied event, when she swam for South Africa at 2002 Commonwealth Games.

Man with no feet is the fastest man in the world and a woman with one leg is one of the fastest swimmers of the world, is a live proof that we are limited only by our imagination.

Lance Conquered Cancer to Make World Record in Cycling

Lance Armstrong (born on September 18, 1971) was diagnosed with lung cancer and brain tumour on October 2, 1996. After curing himself from cancer, he became the first man in the world to win the most gruelling cycling championship 'Tour-de-France' 7 times.

CHAPTER -FOURTEEN

SUPER SPECIALTY HOME HOSPITAL (CONSTRUCTION) STEP -4

It will take less than ₹ 10,000/- and at the most (maximum) 15 days (less than 15 min per day) to build a fully functional Super Specialty Home Hospital. Follow the steps to build your own natural, the most reliable, inexpensive, with no side effects, a high speed healing system.

Step I: The Iron frame: Build an iron frame to hold the required things for complete healing. (Refer page no. 83 for the shape of the frame).

Step II: Collect the following items. Some of the item with "✓" mark are to be placed in the accessory box.

1) Trays (10 x 14 inches)

2) Copper Jug✓

3) Green Lamp✓

4) Ginger✓

5) Lemon✓

6) Garlic✓

7) Amla✓

8) One Kg Pure Honey✓

9) Small Scissors✓

10) Measuring Cup✓

11) pH Strip✓

12) Memory Watch

13) Enema Bag✓

14) Cotton✓

15) Bandage✓

16) Wheat Grass Juicer

17) Imam Dasta (Mortar & Pestle) ✓

18) DVDs of Funny Videos✓

19) Implant Syringe✓

20) Dropper

21) Stress Buster Chart

22) 10 Kgs of Organic Wheat Grains

23) 10 Kgs of Fertile Soil

24) 20 Kgs of Organic Manure

25) Sprouting Bags

26) Musical Science of Belief CD✓

27) 2 Fully Grown Shyama Tulsi Plants

28) Wellness Time Table

29) Rack for Holding 10 Trays

30) The Training Manual (The book 'How to Build a Super Specialty Home Hospital', which you are holding in your hand right now)

(To get a free electronic version of musical Science of Belief CD, funny videos, stress buster chart and wellness time table please send your request at biswaroop@yahoo.com)

Step III: How to Grow Wheat Grass

1) Buy large sized ten (10) trays measuring 10 x 14 inches along with 10 kgs of good quality organic wheat grains.

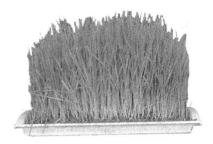

Wheat Grass Tray

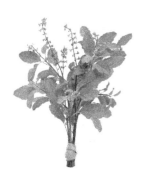

Shyama Tulsi Plant

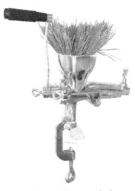

Wheat Grass Juicer

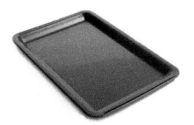

Tray (10x14 inch)

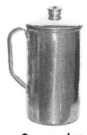

Copper Jug

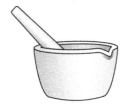

Mortar and Pestle

Points to Keep in Mind While Growing Wheat Grass

a) The weight of wheat grains you take should be accurate in weight according to the instructions.

b) You need soil from a fertile area and organic manure or cow dung as manure. Mix soil as well as manure in 1:2 ratio and spread it on the tray evenly.

c) For measuring, measuring cup should be used given in the kit.

d) For accurate measurement of grains, weighing scale will also be required.

The Steps to Follow for Growing Wheat Grass

1) Step 1, take 100 gm wheat grains (of good quality) and then soak them at least for 12 hours.

2) Step 2, now drain the water after 12 hour from the wheat grains and keep them in sprout bag (for next 12 hour) in order to get sprouted wheats.

3) Step 3, Place a layer of soil in the bottom of the big sized tray about an inch thin (2.4 cms), and then spread a thin layer of sprouted wheat (kept in sprouted bag)over the soil (mixed with manure), i.e next to soil. It should be noticed that seeds should be touching each other, but not overlapping, Next you have to cover the sprouted wheat with a thin layer of soil (mixed with manure) so that the sprouts can be covered properly; this will help to keep the seeds moist.

4) For growing next 9 trays (total trays 10) consecutively, just repeat steps from 1 to 3.

5) Now sprinkle water regularly for at least 7 to 10 days.

6) When your wheatgrass will grow rapidly to about 8 - 10 inches (20 - 24 cms) in 7 to 10 days (if the conditions are good and favorable), then get

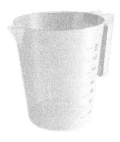

Measuring Cup

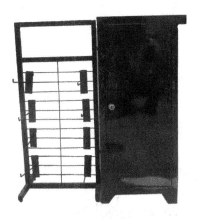

Wheat Grass Rack

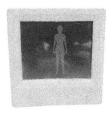

Green Lamp

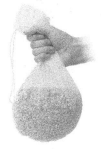

Sprouting Bags

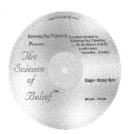

Musical Science of Belief CD

a pair of scissors and cut the wheatgrass from the bottom of the stem as near to the surface as possible.

7) Now extract the juice of the wheat grass with the help of wheat grass juicer. This juice should be taken on an empty stomach, preferably the first thing after getting up in the morning. For maintaining a good health, 50ml of wheat grass juice per day is sufficient. For curing a serious disease 100 ml to 300 ml of wheat grass juice is required to be consumed per day.

Now repeat this process for all 10 trays and enjoy lushy green wheat grass juice.

Now your Super Specialty Home Hospital is ready for use. Remember the S2 H2 is sufficient just for one user at a time. You will be surprised to see that only the above given items are sufficient to literally treat any disease on the earth. And also the success rate and the speed of healing is much higher than the modern day hospitals that too without any side effect. In this S2 H2 you are the patient as well as the doctor. To know how to be your own doctor, go through following chapters.

CHAPTER -FIFTEEN

SUPER SPECIALTY HOME HOSPITAL (APPLICATION) STEP -5

How to use S2 H2?

After 15 days of hard work in collecting all the 28 items needed for the S2 H2 and growing of all the 10 wheat grass trays, now it is ready for use and finally you can say good bye to all the conventional modern medicines, as in many cases getting treated for illness may cost you a fortune and can be **deadlier** than the disease itself.

S2H2 can be used for two purposes:

1) Treating any minor and major illness:-Follow from step 1 to step 5.

2) For overall superior health and fitness. You may skip the first step and start from step 2 to step 5.

Step 1: Repairman (for treating a specific disease)

Step 2: Cleansing of the Body

Step 3: Mental Imagery

Step 4: Super Specialty Master Plan (S2MP)

Step 5: Mastering Any Emotion

Step 1: The Repairman

This section is disease oriented. It is targeted at eliminating specific illness. For this you will be requiring Tulsi, Garlic, Ginger, Lemon, Amla & Honey along with some easy to find kitchen herbs. Patients should follow from Step 1 to Step 5 for a complete cure.

REFERENCE FOR DISEASES

Note: If the name of the disease you are looking for, does not feature in the above list then mail / SMS us for a quick natural cure.
E-mail: biswaroop@yahoo.com Mob.: +91-9312286540

ACIDITY: Apart from human body functioning during digestion, the stomach secretes acid that aids in the breakdown of food. But when the gastric gland of the stomach produces excessive amounts of such acids, it leads to an ailment known as acidity.

Causes:	Symptoms:
• Excessive hot spicy, fried food • Intake of fats, sweets, adulterated and fermented food • Excess smoking	• Burning sensation in the chest and throat • Sour oral secretion/Belching • Bloating, Vomiting and Nausea

Cure:

- It is a natural remedy to drink two glasses of water in the morning regularly. This helps in maintaining the levels of acids in stomach.
- The person suffering from acidity must consume tulsi leaves on a regular basis.
- Chewing a small piece of fresh ginger with salt, five to ten minutes before meals, stimulates digestion.
- Take fresh aloe vera juice in a dose of 10ml to 20ml, two or three times a day. It is an effective cure for acidity.

Juice Therapy:

- The juice of spinach (palak) in its raw state can reduce acidity up to an extent.
- Mango juice should be consumed by people, who have digestion related problems like acidity.
- Drink up to 200 ml of broccoli and spinach juices daily. Juicing is one of the best ways to reduce acidity with vegetables, because it is much easier for the body to assimilate liquids.
- A medium sized cup of raw potato juice taken daily also cures acidity.

ACNE: It is quite common in teenagers. In this, age hormonal changes stimulate glands to produce larger quantities of sebum than before thus, making skin greasier leading to acne.

Causes:	•Symptoms:
• Hormonal changes during puberty	•Pimples
• Secretion of excessive oil in the skin	•Pustules
• High stress levels	•Whiteheads
	•Blackheads
	•Cysts

Cure:
- A teaspoonful of coriander juice, mixed with a pinch of turmeric powder, is another effective remedy for pimples and blackheads. The mixture should be applied to the face after thoroughly washing it, every night before retiring to bed.
- Fresh juice of tender tulsi leaves should be applied externally daily on face.
- Lemon can also play a vital role for acne treatment. First of all boil one litre water to sterilize it. Add freshly squeezed out juice of one lemon to it. Wash and clean the acne- affected area with this water twice daily.
- Intake of amla juice for few days.
- Apply Aloe Vera juice all over the face and keep it for at least 20 minutes and wash it off with luke warm water. Repeat this for at least two weeks.

Juice Therapy:
- Aloe Vera juice is nature's greatest weapon to fight against acne, because it is one of the best ways to detoxify our body. The intake of Aloe Vera juice gives excellent results by purifying the blood.
- Acne is a signal that the organs of excretion aren't functioning optimally. For this the liver can be stimulated with a blend of one part beet root juice, three parts carrot juice and two parts water to help clear the complexion from the inside out.
- Paste of roasted pomegranate is good in treating boils, pimples, blackheads and whiteheads. Apply this paste on the infected parts for at least 15 minutes, and then wash it off with luke-warm water.

ANAEMIA: Anaemia is a health ailment, that takes place as a result of lack of red blood cells or hemoglobin in the body. It's a protein in your red blood cells that carries oxygen from lungs to the rest of your body.

Symptoms:	Causes:
• Dizziness and unconsciousness • Rapid heartbeat • Slow healing of wounds • Pale fingernails, lips and ear lobes	• Low formation of red blood cells due to defects in bone marrow • An inadequate intake of iron • Intestinal parasites

Cure: 50 ml of wheat grass juice twice a day preferably on an empty stomach.

Juice Therapy:

- Strawberries, Broccoli and Citrus juices can help correct nutritional imbalances that lead to Anaemia. Juices high in vitamin C for maximum iron absorption can cure Anaemia.
- Spinach has an excellent ingredient for curing anemia when combined with other ingredients; you would consume rich nutrients to include carotene, vitamins C and E, selenium, zinc, and bioflavonoid. For juice, you can have one half cup fresh spinach, two celery stalks, three carrots, one half lemon and one-half beet on daily basis.

ANOREXIA NERVOSA (LOSS OF APPETITE WITH NERVOUS ANXIETY): This condition is self induced and seen mainly in young women. It is considered to be a psychological disorder which begins with an effort to be thin/slim.

Causes:
- Neurotic personality
- Failure to eat an adequate nutritious diet
- Upset Metabolism

Symptoms:
- Stoppage of menstrual periods
- Impatient, irritable and depressed

Cure:
- Mix 5 ml of lime juice with equal quantity of ginger juice, and 3 ml of honey should be added to this mixture. 2 teaspoon should be taken after each meal everyday.
- 5 gm of ginger should be grounded and licked with little honey after each meals.
- Garlic soup should be taken with lemon juice for better result.

Juice Therapy:
- Oranges are extremely beneficial for anorexia. They stimulate the flow of digestive juices and thus help in improving digestion and appetite. Oranges help to stimulate the production of various digestive juices in the stomach and thus improves your whole digestive system.
- Ginger has certain elements that help you regain your lost appetite. So including a good amount of ginger can help you to come out of your disorder.
- Patients suffering from anorexia are advised to take fruit juices like apples, pears, grapes, oranges, pineapples, peaches at regular intervals.

ARTHRITIS: The word 'arthritis' means 'inflammation of joints'. In this chronic disease one or two joints may become completely deformed, leaving the patient handicapped and weakened. It usually occurs in the older age group.

Causes:	Symptoms:
• Inability to produce endorphin	•Inflammation of the joints
• Joint injuries, infections	•Deformity of joints
• Stress and sprain	•Swelling of joints

Cure:
- Have 1-2 garlic cloves first thing in the morning with water.
- Squeeze half a lemon in one glass of hot water and drink it. Have this 8 to 10 times a day. Initially for few days you might feel that the pain is increasing, but gradually it decreases.
- Drink 50 ml of amla juice for 4 weeks preferably on an empty stomach.

Juice Therapy:
- Black cherry juice is good for arthritis. Patients with arthritis can get relief after drinking two glasses of this juice twice a day.
- Drinking apples juice is good, if you are suffering from arthritis. Apples carry a substantial amount of potassium and have been known to ease arthritis.
- Potato juice has anti-inflammatory actions and reduces excessive deposition of uric acid in the joints in arthritis. Moreover a decoction of clean potato peels or tea made from the peels is recommended also for curing arthritis.

ASTHMA : Asthma is a condition, where respiratory track becomes irritated and inflamed and produces extra mucous .Breathing becomes difficult due to the blockage in wind pipe.

Causes:	Symptoms:
• Allergic conditions like weather, food drugs, perfumes • Allergens like pollen grains, animal hair, fungus and insects, dust etc.	• Tightness in the chest • Profuse sweating and vomiting • Coughing and breathlessness

Cure:

- The patient should fast for a few days on lemon juice with honey.
- The juice of one clove of garlic is mixed with a tsp of honey should be consumed twice a day to dilate the contracted bronchial tubes.
- Tulsi leaves with honey is also beneficial. 1 tsp of tulsi juice and 1 tsp of honey mixed together should be taken 3 times a day.

Juice Therapy:

- In Apple juice, flavanoids and phenolic acids are the ingredients that are beneficial and treat asthma.
- Although Lemon is acidic, but when it enters the body as an acid, it ends up as alkaline residue after your cells use it up. So start taking lemonade everyday to cure Asthma.
- Asthma can also be cured by drinking carrot's root juice daily. Consume at least 20 ml of juice on a regular basis.

BACK PAIN: Back pain is one of the most common problem, we face when our back is over –burdened or strained.

Causes:	Symptoms:
• Weak abdominal and back muscles • Wearing high heels • Long hours of sitting • Lifting heavy loads in an incorrect way	• Pain felt in the middle of the back or in the lower back • In acute stage, the patient is bed ridden and unable to move

Cure:
- Boil water with a few Tulsi leaves and Black Cardamom for drinking.
- Crush 5 Garlic Cloves and add this to a glass of milk. Boil it on a mild flame till ¼ glass remains. Make two equal parts and take 1 part in the morning and 1 part in the evening. This should be repeated for 30 days for better result.
- Direct application of fresh Aloe Vera gel on back provides an instant relief.

Juice Therapy:
- Lemon juice has always been considered to be one of the best and quickest cures for back pain. Lemon juice contains vitamin C, which has been proven to reduce and eliminate back pain.
- Cherry juice contains anti-inflammatory properties that aid in reducing back pain.

Note : Lemon juice is highly acidic and can cause pitting of the tooth enamel. Rinse your mouth thoroughly after you drink lemon juice to protect your teeth from enamel corrosion.

BAD BREATH OR HALITOSIS: It's a dental condition which causes bad breath and gum conditions.

Causes:

- In halitosis or bad breath, dental decay of the teeth may result in abscesses in the gum with foul smelling, pus giving an objectionable odour to the breath. Even small holes in the teeth may provide a place where germs can multiply and release foul odour
- Smoking

Symptoms:
- Odorous breath
- An unpleasant taste in the mouth
- Improper cleaning of teeth

Cure:

- Chewing four or five leaves of Tulsi two to four times a day especially after meals, will clean the mouth, remove bad odours emanating from the mouth and get rid of a bad taste in the mouth. A regular use of Tulsi will in fact cure all disorders of the mouth.
- Gargling with a decoction of Tulsi plant provides protection from disorders of the teeth such as decay, cures any disease of the teeth that has been contracted previously, and kills the micro-organism infesting the teeth.
- Drink water throughout the day to keep your mouth moistened. A dry mouth will be more likely to cause bad breath.
- Chew a little amount of wheatgrass for 3 to 5 minutes a day.

Juice Therapy:
- Daily intake of Pineapple Juice vanishes bad breath up to large extent.
- Apple juice also helps in removing bad breath and is good for mouth purification, as it removes the bacteria causing bad breath.
- Wheat grass juice helps to reduce the strong odor and is an excellent source of chlorophyll, which helps in removing bad breath.

BED WETTING : Bed wetting means involuntary urination on bed at night. This condition is more common in children. Children generally after the age of 3-4 gain control over the bladder, but in some children, this mechanism some how is not strengthened and they pass urine in bed subconsciously.

Causes:
- Infection in the urinary bladder
- Worms in stool & intestine
- Emotional immaturity

Symptoms:
- No control over the bladder functions specially at night

Cure:
- A teaspoonful of pure honey should be given to the child, before going to the bed.
- Eating one teaspoon of raisins and two teaspoon of walnut halves can help to combat the problem of bed wetting.

Juice Therapy:
- Consume one medium glass of cranberry (karaunda) juice, one hour before going to bed,
- You can use celery juice on daily basis in order to avoid bed wetting.

BOILS: Boils are painful, red, pus filled swelling in the skin surrounded by large red areas. These are caused by type of bacterias that live silently on the surface of the skin.

Causes:	Symptoms:
• Boils are caused by bacteria which enter the sweat gland or hair follicles • Sometime caused by blood impurities also • Faulty diets and wrong style of living	• Boils occur on face, eyelids, back of the neck, upper back and buttocks • Painful red nodules appear on the skin

Cure:

• The juice of Garlic can be applied externally on the boils to help them ripen and also to break them and to evacuate the pus.

• Warm moist compress should be applied three to four times a day over the tender areas. This will help to bring the boil to a burst and encourage easy drainage of pus.

• Aloe Vera gel is excellent to ease burns, relieve inflammation and accelerate healing. Aloe Vera gel has anti-fungal, anti-bacterial and anti-viral properties. It lessens painful effects of burns.

Juice Therapy:

• Like many other skin ailments, boils result from a build-up of toxins in the system. To stimulate the liver and speed up the elimination of wastes, drink a blend of Carrot, Beet Root, and Celery juice. A large glass in morning and a smaller glass in the afternoon is an effective and a very nutritious way to heal the boils.

BRONCHITIS: It is a breathing disorder, affecting the respiratory function. It occurs when the wind pipe is blocked with mucous caused by infection etc. This causes acute coughing and breathing difficulties.

Causes:	Symptoms:
•Cigarette smoking •Dust and air pollution	• Severe cough especially during the morning of winter months • Tightness around the chest • Breathlessness on exertion • Wheezing or whistling sound while breathing

Cure:
- The juice of Ginger (1 teaspoon) mixed with honey should be taken thrice a day.
- The decoction of Tulsi, Ginger and Black pepper in equal quantities taken three times a day.
- Mix 1 teaspoon Garlic pulp and 3 teaspoons honey and consume it three times a day.
- Drinking 50 ml of Amla juice for 1 month.

Juice Therapy:
- Juices rich in the antioxidant nutrients beta-carotene and vitamin C strengthen the immune system. Even vegetable sugar has been shown to boost the immune system. For this use three Broccoli florets and a clove of garlic with four or five carrots, two celery stalks and half of a capsicum. To shore up the immune system, drink this blend several times a day.
- Turnip juice mixed with Cabbage orCcarrot juice, taken daily reduces mucous and helps in curing bronchitis.

BURNS: A burn is damage to your body's skin surface and tissue.

Causes:	Symptoms:
• Heat • Chemicals • Electricity • Sunlight or Radiation	• Immediate redness of skin • Burn leaves a painless white or charred area

Cure:

• Pain due to burns is alleviated by applying equal quantities of tulsi juice and coconut oil mixed well. Tulsi alone can also work for burns.

• If it is a burn from hot liquids then rub the affected area immediately with ice cubes and then apply a solution of milk and honey. This prevents formation of blisters.

• For slight burns the application of honey will reduce the burning sensation.

• Sliced potatoes can also be used on an effected area for relief.

• Aloe Vera gel is excellent to ease burns, relieve inflammation and accelerate healing. Aloe vera gel has anti-fungal, anti-bacterial and anti-viral properties. It lessens painful effects of burns.

Juice Therapy:

•Papaya contains enzymes that help to remove dead cells from the wound. So have papaya juice daily.

•Carrot juice also helps in healing burns. For that apply carrot juice directly on the effective parts.

HIGH CHOLESTEROL: Cholesterol a yellowish fatty substance, although it is essential to life, upto some extent, but it has a bad reputation, being a major villain in heart diseases.

Causes:	Symptoms:
• Excessive consumption of milk and its products like ghee, butter and cream • Irregularity in habits, smoking, drinking alcohols • Fried food and oily food	• High cholesterol doesn't have any symptom, for that you go through a simple blood test called a Lipoprotein Profile

Cure:
- Person with a high cholesterol should drink at least 8 to 10 glasses of water every day. As regular drinking of water stimulates the excretory activity of the skin and kidneys.
- Regular drinking of coriander water is beneficial too. To prepare it we need dry seeds of coriander and straining the decoction after boiling it with water.
- Increase the intake of raw Garlic boiled in water, as it helps to reduce the Cholesterol.
- Intake of aloe vera juice, results in marked reduction of fats in body, so this juice is quite helpful in high cholesterol.

Juice Therapy:
- Beet root juice is considered to be one of the most powerful cleansers of the body. It is rich in Vitamin A, Sodium, Calcium, Chlorine, Vitamin B6, Sulfur, Iron, and Potassium.
- Consume Lemon juice and 1 tsp Honey in luke-warm glass of water with empty stomach in morning and at night.

Note: Pure raw beet root juice may increase your heart rate. So to decrease side effects, it is suggested to mix beet root juice with other fruits or vegetables, e.g. apples, carrots, cucumbers etc.

CATARACT: Opacification of the lens of the eye or its capsule (covering) sufficient to interfere with vision is called cataract.

Causes:	Symptoms:
• Malnutrition • Vitamin A or B deficiency • Diabetes • Old age • Infection of an eye	• Patients complain of blurring of vision in the early stages of the disease • Complete vision is impaired in the affected eye at later stage

Cure:

• Mix 1 teaspoon Rose water (Gulab Jal) with 1 teaspoon fresh Lemon juice. Put 1 drop twice or thrice to the affected eye.

Juice Therapy:

• Juices rich in beta-carotene and Vitamin C can slowdown the development of cataract. These nutrients protect the eye from free radical damage caused by exposure to the Sun. Take out juice of two celery stalks and four or five carrots. Drinking this juice will help in protecting your eyes from further damage.

• Person suffering from cataract should take plenty of raw Carrots daily, two glasses of fresh Carrot juice should be taken, one each in the morning and evening.

COLD : There is no cure for prevention of cold. It is relieved naturally within a week. The cold is treated by attempting to relieve its symptom such as head ache, stuffy nose and congestion.

Causes:	Symptoms:
• Wrong food habits	• Sneezing
• Cold can occur due to 200 or more viruses	• Watery eyes
• Viral infection	• Sore throat
• Sudden change in temperature	• Cough and hoarseness
• Long exposure to a cold environment	• Runny nose
	• Chilling of the body

Cure:
- Eat one Amla twice a day.
- The juice of two Lemons in ½ litre of boiling water sweetened with honey, taken at bed time is a very effective remedy.
- Take two teaspoonfuls of tulsi juice and two teaspoonfuls of Ginger juice with Honey every morning and evening.

Juice Therapy :
- Orange juice is good in case of cold. Orange juice contains high levels of vitamin C.
- Squeezing a lemon into a glass of water is also recommended and adding a spoon of honey will help to increase its effectiveness and palatability.
- Fresh mixed vegetable juice for a cold is commonly used to help in decreasing the length of the recovery period.

CONSTIPATION: Constipation is a common disturbance of the digestive tract. People who are constipated may find it difficult and painful to have regular bowel movement.

Causes:	Symptoms:
• Insufficient fibre in diet • Less fluid intake • Reasonable time should be given for passing stool. (Most of the people because of a fast life schedule give very less time for proper defecation)	• Bloated feeling in the stomach, discomfort, general unease due to gas • Irregularity or difficulty of elimination due to hard feceal matter • Pimple on the face • Dark circle under the eyes

Cure:

• Drinking water which has been kept overnight in a copper vessel, the first thing in the morning will bring good results.

• Drinking hot water with 1 teaspoon honey and juice of ½ a lemon first thing in the morning.

• Drinking one litre water in the morning in one go.

• The deposition of toxins and unwanted substances in our diet which keep accumulating in intestines prevent the absorption of essential nutrients causing nutritional deficiency, , causes constipation. Aloe juice helps in flushing out these residues boosting the digestion and giving a greater feeling of well-being.

Juice Therapy:

• Start the day with blend of equal parts Apple, BeetRroot and Carrot, along with 1 tsp of ginger juice. Apple juice contains sorbitol, a natural sugar with laxative properties, which help in treating constipation.

• Folate deficiency can also aggravate constipation, juicing dark green leafy vegetables such as spinach and asparagus, are excellent sources of this nutrient, it prevents constipation.

• Pumpkin juice is really a good natural remedy for constipation. It is an excellent stool softener.

• Raw cucumber juice is an effective laxative that aids bowel action and removes constipation.

• Prune (alubukhara) juice, a natural laxative, can also be consumed every day to prevent constipation. Prune juice may taste better, if mixed with another juice, such as apple and apricot (khumani). Apple and apricot juice also help in soften stools.

•

Note:
• Sticky foods like banana and yogurt (curd) should be avoided. Banana is responsible for constipation, so avoid taking banana in constipation.

COUGH: The air passage of the lungs are lined with cells secreting mucous, which normally traps particles of dust. When the membranes are infected and inflamed, the secretion of mucous increases and the lining of air pessage is irritated.

Causes:	**Symptoms:**
• Consumption of cold or sour food by people with sensitive throats	• Generally cough is worse in the morning, it brings up some thick yellow or green phlegm
• Cough may be caused by clogging of the bronchial tube with waste matter	

Cure:
• 5 fresh Tulsi leaves well mixed in 10 ml of pure honey, chewed twice a day, calms down cough in children and adults .
• 5 ml of fresh onion juice well mixed with 10 ml of pure honey should be taken twice a day for 10 days.
• To stay away from all kind of cough, boil some fresh basil leaves in water. Drink this water every morning.
• Mix equal amounts of honey and ginger (adrak) juice. For better result have 1 teaspoon 2-3-4 times a day.

Juice Therapy:
• Grapes are one of the most effective home remedies for the treatment of a Cough. Grapes tone up the lungs and act as an expectorant, relieving a simple cough in a couple of days. A cup of

Grape juice mixed with a teaspoon of Honey is advised for Cough relief.

- The juice of raw onion is valuable in a Cough. One teaspoon of the juice should be mixed with one teaspoon of honey and kept for four or five hours. It will make an excellent Cough syrup and should be taken twice daily.
- In the case of a severe cough, the patient should fast on orange juice and water till the severity is reduced. The procedure is to take the juice of an Orange diluted in a cup of warm water, every two hours from 8 a.m. to 8 p.m.

CHOLERA: Cholera is one of the most severe diseases of the intestine. It is water borne disease and common during the monsoons.

Causes:	Symptoms:
• Caused by rod shaped germ known as Vibrio Cholerae • Incorrect eating habits and faulty style of living	• Upset stomach • Vomitting and fever in early stage. • Terrible muscles and stomach cramp

Cure:
- The juice of lemon can kill virus in a short span of time, moreover daily intake of lemon with food can also prevent Cholera.
- Boil a few basil leaves and strain the decoction, cool it down and have it once a day.

Juice Therapy:
- Make a blend of 30 grams of Onion Juice with 10 Black Peppers. Consume this twice a day.
- A glass of Orange juice is highly effective, on a daily basis to cure Cholera.

DANDRUFF: Dandruff is the harmless disease of the skin/scalp. It is the excessive flaking of dead skin that forms on the scalp.

Causes:	Symptoms:
• It can be due to too much or too little oil being produced by sebaceous glands in the scalp • Fungal infection of the scalp	• Scaliness increases whenever the hair is brushed • With Itching scalp may become red from scratching • Falling of dandruff constantly

Cure:

- About 25 gm of dry Amla is soaked in a litre of water overnight. It is boiled in the morning, until half of it remains. To this 25 gm of yoghurt is added and this paste should be applied on the scalp. After one hour of the paste, the scalp should be washed first with Amla water and then with plain water, This procedure should be repeated every week for 2 to 3 months.
- A few drops of Lime juice mixed with amla juice should be applied to scalp every night, before going to bed.
- Apply fresh Aloe Vera juice on the scalp and message gently. Wait for 30 minutes and rinse well with water.

Juice Therapy:

- The juice of Snake Gourd (chichinda/padval) has been found beneficial in the prevention and treatment of dandruff. The juice should be rubbed over the scalp for this purpose.
- Dandruff can be removed by massaging the hair for half an hour with curd or with a few drops of Lime juice mixed with Amla juice every night, before going to bed.

DEHYDRATION : Loss of water or insufficient water level in the body leads to dehydration.

Causes:	Symptoms:
•Excessive vomiting, Diarrhea	• Acute weakness

Cure:
- Lemon juice and honey can be mixed well. Drink this 5 to 6 times a day.

Juice Therapy:
- Watermelon is a particularly good choice for curing dehydration, because of high water content.
- Lime juice provides quick hydration and rejuvenation, just by drinking a glass of lime juice. It is good to fight fatigue as well as vomiting bouts.
- Drink a mixture of 1 tsp mint juice, 1/2 tsp Ginger juice and 1 tsp Honey three times a day.
- For curing dehydration, increase the intake of Papaya, Apple, Pomegranate, Carrot, Potato juices.
- Eat one green Banana, after every two to four hour, until the symptoms subside.

DEPRESSION: Depression is the most prevalent of all the emotional disorders. This may vary from feeling of slight sadness to utter misery and dejection.

Causes:	Symptoms:
• Depleted functioning of the adrenal glands	• Acute sense of loss
• The excessive and indiscriminate use of drugs	• Inexplicable sadness
	• Loss of energy
• Excessive use of Aspirin	• Lack interest in world

Cure:
- Have an Apple with Milk and Honey.
- Add Rose petals in a glass of boiling water. Add sugar to the drink. Cool it and have it.
- Drinking 10-30ml of Aloe Vera juice with empty stomach at morning is quite beneficial in curing depression.

Juice Therapy:
- Apple juice is one of the most valuable remedies for mental depression. The various chemical substances present in this fruit such as vitamin B, phosphorus, and potassium help the synthesis of glutamic acid, which controls the wear and tear of nerve cells. This remedy will act as a very effective nerve tonic and recharge the nerves with new energy and life.
- Wheat Grass juice is also recommended for curing depression. Consume 50 ml of wheat grass juice with empty stomach in the morning.
- According to a recent survey conducted by MIND amongst people suffering from depression, many felt much better after having Banana pulp juice. This is because Bananas contain tryptophan, a type of protein that the body converts into serotonin known to make you relax, improve your mood and generally make you feel happier.

DIABETES: A disease in which the body does not produce or properly use insulin (a hormone that is needed to convert sugar, starches and other food into energy needed for daily life).

Causes:	Symptoms:
• Genetic factor	• Unusual thirst
• Excessive consumption of alcohol	• Frequent urination
• Over weight	• Reducing vision
• Excessive use of sugar and fats	• Itching and boils

Cure:
• Chew 10-15 Basil leaves in the morning.
• A tablespoon of Amla juice mixed with honey can be taken daily as a dose.
• A glass of lukewarm water with freshly squeezed Lemon juice can be taken.
• Consume 10-30ml of aloe vera juice daily with empty stomach at morning & 30 minutes before dinner at night.

Juice Therapy:
• Gooseberry (Amla), with its high vitamin C content, is considered valuable in diabetes. A tablespoon of its juice, mixed with a cup of Bitter Gourd juice, should be taken daily for two months. This mixture will reduce the blood sugar in Diabetes.
• French Beans are very effective for people having diabetes as the juice of the French Beans stimulates the production of insulin. It can be taken along with Cabbage juice.
• Equal quantities of amla juice and Bitter Gourd (Karela) juice taken every morning also reduce blood glucose levels.
• A person should consume Pear juice, as they contain levulose a fruit sugar more easily tolerated by people with diabetes.

DIARRHOEA: Diarrhoea refers to the frequent passage of loose or watery unformed stool. It can be acute or chronic. Commonly known as "loose motion". It is perhaps the most common disease in India.

Causes:	Symptoms:
• Overeating or eating of wrong food.	• Anaemic and pale face
• Infection in the intestinal tract	• Abdominal pain
• Use of antibiotic drugs and excessive intake of laxatives.	• Nausea and vomiting

Cure:
• Mix little salt in juice of Lemon, drink it without diluting with water.
• Swallow 25 grams of powdered Tulsi seeds with 10 ml of Honey.

Juice Therapy:
• Carrot juice is another effective home remedy for Diarrhea. It supplies water to combat dehydration. It also checks the growth of harmful intestinal bacteria and prevents vomiting. Carrot juice should be given in small amounts to the patient every half an hour.
• Capsicum is a stimulant herb. It's juice helps in relieving gastrointestinal problems like Diarrhea.
• Potato juice mixed with carrot and pure honey will disinfect the bowels in case of any food poisoning and this also stops Diarrhea.

DYSENTERY: Dysentery is a serious condition affecting the large intestine. In other words it is the infection of the digestive tract.

Causes:	Symptoms:
• Germ infection • Over spiced food • Excessive amount of flesh food	• Poor appetite • Pain in the lower abdomen before passing stool • Onset is usually abrupt with high fever, followed by vomiting, abdominal pain. • Stool sometime tinged with blood

Cure:

• 50 gm Yoghurt mixed with small amount of honey should be taken 3 times a day.
• A few pieces of peeled and sliced Lemon, should be added to 250 ml of water and boiled for a few minutes, a strained decoction should be taken thrice.

Juice Therapy:

• Fresh berries (ber) rejuvenate the pancreas, and their antiseptic value helps in relieving dysentery.
• Lemon juice is also quite effective in ordinary cases of dysentery.

Note: Those who suffer from Diarrhea or dysentery should restrict the consumption of leafy vegetables.

ECZEMA: Eczema means boiling over of the skin and is characterized by spontaneous eruption ranging from mild to severe. In chronic cases, the skin becomes thickened and appears like the bark of a tree.

Causes:	Symptoms:
• Allergic reaction with pesticides, astringent, perfumes, harsh soaps, detergents and household cleaner • Inherited stress • Allergies to dust, pollen etc	• Bleeding on skin surface. • Pus or other discharge • Itchiness

Cure:

• Apply crushed Garlic directly on the affected areas.
• Apply aloe vera gel directly on the effected parts, three times a day in beginning and then reduce the application accordingly.

Juice Therapy:

• Fresh juice of apricots (Khumani) is good for curing eczema. Drink 50 ml of apricot juice for 15 days.

• Consumption of Wheatgrass juice is effective against eczema. Chlorophyll in Wheatgrass juice is an excellent detoxifying agent. It also helps in the maintenance of acidity or alkalinity levels. Enzymes in the juice enhance the immune system.

PUS IN THE EAR : Pus in the ear occurs due to inflammation of the ear which is caused by certain bacterias and viruses.

Causes:	Symptoms:
• Pus in the ear is due to cough, cold and sinusitis • Entrance of bacteria into the middle ear • Infection of the ear	• When the pus is formed in the middle ear, child complains of severe pain in the ear which is unbearable. • Vomiting, poor appetite, cough. • In most cases the pus enters into the external ear and outside after the eardrum is ruptured.

Cure:
- In the case of pus inside the ear, warm 1 tbsp onion juice on fire and put 2-3 drops into the ears 2 to 3 times a day. For Onion juice, Grate onion and squeeze well to take out the juice.
- Mix a Clove of Garlic into 1 tbsp of olive oil, put it into the ear after sieving the mixture.
- Onion juice is very effective in treating any ear infections. For this purpose prepare Onion juice and put two to three drops of it in the affected ear.
- Prepare juice form fresh holy basil leaves and put few drops of this juice in your infected ear.

Juice Therapy:
- Drinking mix vegetables and fruit juices are the best way to cure ear infection very fast.

GOUTY PAINS: A painful form of arthritis which affect the big toe, ankle, knee, foot, hand, elbow and wrist. Men are at least 4 times more likely to develop gout than women.

Causes :	Symptoms:
• Excess uric acid in the body results in crystalline deposits in the joints • It can be hereditary disease • Excessive intake of alcohol	• Painful swelling of the joint and acute pain in big toe • Redness and tenderness of the joint area • The attack usually occurs at midnight or in the early hours of the morning

Cure:
- Just squeeze half Lemon in a glass of warm water, add a little honey and drink in the morning.
- Add half a teaspoon of Baking Soda in a glass of water and drink it to alleviate Gout Pain.

Juice Therapy:
- The fresh Cherry juice is considered effective in treating Gout. Consume about fifteen to twenty Cherrie's juice a day, preferably as soon as you wake up. Subsequently, you can begin to reduce the amount of Cherries you consume. Research into the effectiveness of cherries for treating gout showed that an antioxidant in cherries called anthocyanins helps to relieve inflammation as well as reduce the frequency of Gout flare-ups.
- Apples are regarded as an excellent source for curing Gout. The malic acid in them is believed to neutralize the uric acid providing relief to gout sufferers. The patient is advised to take one Apple juice after each meal.
- Bananas have been found beneficial in the treatment of Gout. Diet of bananas only for three or four days is advised for providing some relief from gout. A patient can take eight or nine banana's pulp juice daily during this period.
- Vitamin C in lemon is known to prevent and cure sore joints by

strengthening the connective tissues of the body. The citric acid found in lime is a solvent of the uric acid, which is the primary cause of this disease. The juice of half a Lime, squeezed into a glass of water, should be taken twice daily.

EPILEPSY : Epilepsy refers to a disorder in which a person has a tendency to have fits. Fit is due to abnormal electrical activity of the brain.

Causes:	Symptoms:
• Injury to baby during delivery	• Patient lose control of urine and stool
• Delay in delivery with decreased oxygen supply to brain.	• After gaining consciousness, the patient may have headache and go to sleep
• Hydrocephalus –excessive fluid in the brain.	• Sudden spasms of head and trunk

Cure:
• Apply fresh lemon juice on the head, massage well before washing off.
• Garlic concoction can be taken for this. Take 3 to 4 Garlic cloves and crush them and boil it with 100ml milk.When reduced to half, it is ready to use.
• Rub Tulsi juice over your body everyday after taking bath. This is very beneficial remedy.

Juice Therapy:
• Consume 20 to 30 ml of wheat grass juice daily on empty stomach.

INSOMNIA: Inability to sleep is called insomnia. Sleep is an essential requirement, as it restores energy and permits us to lead a healthy life.

Causes:	Symptoms:
• Excessive fatigue post illness • Stress and mental tension • Smoking	• Dramatic changes in the duration and quality of sleep • Lapse of memory and lack of concentration during the day

Cure:

• Add 2 teaspoons of honey to a big cup of water and have it before going to bed. Babies generally fall asleep after having honey.

• Raw onions should be eaten daily, with each meal as it induces sound sleep.

• Raw pumpkin juice is rich in magnesium which is a really good sleep inducer as it helps your muscles to relax.

• Honey is a traditional remedy for insomnia. It slightly raises your sugar level in the blood. As a result, the level of insulin increases and helps tryptophan to be absorbed and converted to melanin. It makes you feel relaxed and you can enjoy healthy and restorative sleep.

Juice Therapy:

• Take a glass of pumpkin juice with honey before going to bed and it will give you a good sleep.

HAIR FALL AND LOSS: Hair fall at an early age of life can be very embarrassing especially for young girls and boy's who develop a feeling of social stigma.

Causes:	Symptoms:
• Inadequate nutrition • Deficiency of vitamin and folic acid • Stress, worry and anxiety are also some of the factors	• Thinning of the hair • Constant shedding of hair

Cure:
• Cut a lemon into two halves and massage the scalp, ensuring that you use both the juice and rind while massaging. After half an hour rinse the hair with cold water. Frequent massage with lemon helps in the prevention of hair loss.

Juice Therapy:
• Juice of broccoli and carrot juice is very beneficial in preventing hair fall and loss.

HEADACHE : Pain in the head is often nature's warning that something is wrong somewhere in the body.

Causes:	Symptoms:
• Poor eyesight, fever and injury • High blood pressure	• Throbbing pain between the eyes and in the head • Nausea and dizziness

Cure:
• Consume an apple every morning on empty stomach.
• Fine paste of Cinnamon should be prepared by mixing it with water, and should be applied on temples and forehead to obtain relief.
• For head ache, you can message aloe vera gel gently over the head and keep it for half an hour, then wash it off with water.

Juice Therapy:
• The most common causes of headaches are constipation and liver malfunction. A relief from headache can be obtained from the Grape juice. Grind fresh grapes and drink without adding any water.
• Drink a glass of Celery juice, if you are having head ache. Celery juice is a superb nerve tonic. Celery juice alone tastes a little bitter and is usually mixed with carrots or Apples.

HEART PROBLEM: Heart disease refers to chest pain produced due to increased work by the heart. A reduction in the flow of blood leads to chest pain and heart attack.

Causes:	Symptoms:
• Excessive smoking	• Pain in chest either on the left, centre or even on the right side
• Hypertension	
• Increased blood cholesterol level.	• Difficulty in breathing
• Diabetes	• Sweating is seen in acute attacks
• Lack of exercise	
• Excessive alcohol consumption	• Irregular heart beat, may be seen in some cases
	• Fatigue without valid reason.

Cure:

• One clove of garlic should be taken daily on empty stomach.

• One teaspoon of raw onions juice first thing in the morning will be highly beneficial in such cases.

• One tablespoon honey daily after food is sufficient to prevent all sorts of heart troubles.

Juice Therapy:

• Beet root juice is helpful in treating heart problem, so for this consume 50 ml on daily basis.

• Freshly prepared grape juice is also beneficial for heart, as it tones the heart.

• Apple has heart stimulating properties, so fresh apple juice is also good for curing heart problem.

HEPATITIS: Inflammation of the liver is known as Hepatitis in medical language. This inflammation makes the liver stop working.

Causes:	Symptoms:
• Alcohol or certain drugs	• Flu like illness, nausea and vomiting • Loss of appetite • Weight loss, jaundice • Itchy skin

Cure:

• 1 or 2 teaspoon fresh juice of Coriander leaves mixed in 1 cup buttermilk should be taken 2-3 times.

• Consumption of aloe vera juice has been shown to have beneficial effects on liver in chronic hepatitis patients. So drink 30 ml of AloeVera juice for at least 2 weeks.

Juice Therapy:

• For hepatitis, Beet Root and Carrot juice is preferred on daily basis.

• Wheatgrass juice is quite effective in hepatitis, as it increases immunity at a high speed.

INTESTINAL WORMS: Worms and other intestinal parasites which infest human beings are found in all countries of the world. Children are more infested with these worms than adults.

Causes:	Symptoms:
• Undercooked meat • Dirty fingers and food • Through the skin from infected water • Undercooked flesh food or foods contaminated by dogs	• Diarrhea • Foul smell • Dark circles under eyes. • Constant desire for food • Loss of weight • Nervousness and irritability

Cure:

• Regular use of garlic can be used for expelling intestinal worms.

• Drinking Aloe Vera juice twice a day helps in destroying intestinal worms. It has an alkalinizing and anti-inflammatory effect.

Juice Therapy:

- Pumpkin Juice works very powerfully to push out worms from the digestive tract. No other vegetable or fruit contains as much Vitamin B as the pumpkin.

- Papaya juice is helpful in expelling round worms from the digestive tract. In cases, where patients have taken a course of antibiotics, papaya is recommended to hasten the restoration of friendly symbiotic bacteria in the gut which would have been destroyed by drugs. Papaya cleanses the body completely.

- Intestinal worm's growth in the stomach can be subsided by drinking one tsp mint juice three times a day.

CANCER: Cancer occurs when cell in certain tissue multiply uncontrollably and most commonly affects lungs, bowel, skin, stomach, ovaries, pancreas, prostrate, bladder, breast and lymph gland.

Causes:	Symptoms:
• Genetic disposition	• Unexplained, persistent weight loss
• Heavy drinking	• A mole that changes shape, gets bigger, itches or bleed
• Smoking	• Sores, scabs or ulcer on the skin that do not heal
• Chemical and food additives	• Change in the shape and size of testicles
• Processed and smoked food	• Unexplained severe headache
• Diet high in red meat and other food containing saturated animal fats.	• Persistent abdominal pain or indigestion
• Unprotected sex	• Blood –either red or black –in the stool or urine
• Repressed emotion or lack of spiritual development	• Change in bowel habits e.g constipation for no obvious reasons
	• Vaginal bleeding between menstrual periods or after the menupause

Cure:
- For cancer patients, cantaloupes are quite good; one average-sized cantaloupe contains approximately 100 calories.

Juice Therapy:
- Potato juice can be used in the treatment of cancer and daily intake of potato juice shows a drastic change.
- Abnormal growths, Cancer, Tumors, Ulcers and Fibrous masses seem to be dissolved by the powerful chemical agent in the Grape. So grape juice intake also has been found a panacea for the cancer patients.
- Wheat Grass Juice and Super Specialty Master Plan

INDIGESTION: Our digestive system breaks up all that we eat or drink in useful components, which the body requires to lead a healthy life. Any disturbance in this system leads to indigestion.

Causes:	Symptoms:
• Eating too fast, especially high fat food	• Burning sensation in stomach or chest
• Excessive acid accumulation in the stomach	• Bloating, nausea and burping
• Over consumption of alcohol	
• Stress during pregnancy	

Cure:
- Before eating a heavy meal, one should eat 2 to 3 small pieces of Ginger
- Mix 1 teaspoon of Ginger juice and 1 teaspoon of Lemon juice. Honey can be added according to taste.
- Put 2 to 3 tender leaves of Tulsi in a glass of water overnight and drink this water early in the morning. This will clean your bowels and purify your blood.
- Drink 1 glass of hot water mixed with 2 teaspoon Ginger juice and 1 teaspoon honey.

Juice Therapy:
- Carrot and Cabbage, eliminates indigestion, 3 Carrots, 1/2 head of

cabbage juice is recommended for improving digestion.

- Juicing a slice of fresh ginger, half of a handful of fresh mint, one kiwifruit and one-fourth of a pineapple. Drinking 40 ml blend twice daily, should speed up digestion, soothe the intestine and help in eliminating gas.
- One medium glass of pineapple juice taken after every meal is highly beneficial in indigestion treatment.
- Add a spoonful of lemon juice, one spoonful of ginger and two spoons of honey in a glass of lukewarm water. Mix them well and drink, if indigestion problem occur.
- An orange juice is an effective indigestion remedy, as it gives rest to the digestive organs and supplies nutrition.
- Grapes juice is also effective in removing indigestion and irritation from the stomach.
- Lemon juice helps in curing indigestion, as it fights against bacteria. Consume a tablespoon of lemon juice in a cup of hot water before a meal to prevent acid indigestion.

TOOTH ACHE: Toothache is a most common complaint. Teeth are prone to infections as these are overused and exposed to a variety of

Causes:	Symptoms:
<ul><li>Decay of teeth</li><li>Over-indulgence in sweets</li></ul>	<ul><li>Pain may be constant throughout the day and night</li><li>Severe headache may also follow</li></ul>

Cure:

- A paste prepared from one or two Garlic cloves should be applied on the affected tooth.
- A small piece of onion can also be placed on the affected area.
- Powder 3 cloves of garlic with 1 teaspoon Lemon juice. Apply this on the painful gum and tooth and massage lightly.

Juice Therapy:

- For toothache use onion or Garlic juice. Soak cotton wool in either of these can be used to plug and disinfect the cavity. It is highly beneficial in curing all type of teeth problems.

- Brinjal juice is found to be an effective remedy for Tooth ache. Apply juice of the Brinjal on the effected tooth.

JAUNDICE: Jaundice is the most common of all liver disorders resulting from obstruction in the bile duct.

Causes:	Symptoms:
• Stones in liver	• Yellow complexion
• Blocking the pathway of bile	• Nausea
• Contaminated food and water	• Fatigue and itching
• Certain vitamins deficiency	• Slow pulse
• Liver malfunctioning	• Yellow eye
	• Loss of appetite

Cure:
- Frequently drink Lemon juice
- Plenty of Wheatgrass juice can be given to the patient, to promote more urination as well as for nutrition and general health.
- 1 teaspoon Ginger juice with 1 teaspoon each fresh Lime and Tulsi juice mixed with a tablespoon of honey, should be taken frequently.

Juice Therapy:

- Sugarcane, Papaya & Pineapple juices are excellent in jaundice. Use as much juices as you can and have early recovery.

- Tomatoes are valuable in Jaundice. A glass of fresh Tomato juice, mixed with a pinch of salt and Black Pepper, taken early in the morning, is considered an effective remedy for this disease.

- One glass of Sugarcane juice, mixed with the juice of half a lime, and taken twice daily, can hasten recovery from Jaundice.

INFLAMMATION OF THE GUMS: Swollen or bleeding gums are symptoms of inflammation of the gums.

Causes:	Symptoms:
• Poor oral hygiene • Not cleaning mouth after intake of food	• Difficulty while chewing food • Bleeding and pain in the gums • Teeth fall out one by one

Cure:
• Garlic paste prepared by one or two garlic cloves should be applied on the affected tooth.
• Chewing tulsi leaves after meals can help you out.

Juice Therapy:

• Cranberry (Karounda) juice has shown to help treat and reduces gum diseases. Naturally made vegetable juices contain several vitamins and nutrients that help fight gum disease causing bacteria. Adding grapes to the mixture can improve its taste.

• Wheat grass juice is quite helpful in preventing bacterial growth.

Note: Cranberry may help in curing gum diseases by preventing bacteria from sticking to teeth.

TYPHOID: It is condition in which there is a typical course of temperature, with marked abdominal symptoms consisting of ulceration of the bowels. The fever is of uncertain duration and liable to frequent relapses.

• **Causes:**	**Symptoms:**
• Poor sanitation	• Patient feels chilly, tired and weak
• Contaminated water	• Headache and loss of appetite
• Infected milk	• Back- pain and Diarrhea or constipation

Cure:

• Lemons juice of two or three lemons may be taken each day.

Juice Therapy:

• Garlic juice is good, for curing Typhoid because it contains a lot of iodine which helps people who suffer from hyperthyroidism.

• The skin of pomegranates are rich in the fibres, nutrients and minerals vital to alleviate diarrhea (diarrhea is one of the by-products of typhoid), so the pomegranate juice is preferred in case of typhoid.

KIDNEY STONES: The formation of stones in the kidneys or urinary tract is a fairly common disorder.

Causes	Symptoms:
• Defects in the general metabolism	• Obstruction of flow of urine and pain
• Insufficient intake of fluids	• A desire to urinate frequently
• Excess intake of acid forming foods	• Painful urination
	• Scanty urination

Cure:

- Frequent intake of coriander tea. Boil 2 tsp finely grounded coriander seeds in a glass of boiling hot water. Add honey to taste.
- Basil juice and honey mixed, should be taken for 6 months.

Juice Therapy:

- If you are feeling stones in your kidney, use coconut water. Coconut water is helpful in passing off small stones through urine.
- Banana pulp juice helps in removing kidneys stones. Due to the high potassium content of bananas, a normal intake of potassium suppresses calcium excretion in the urine and minimizes the risk of kidney stones.
- Watermelon Juice is very good fruit for people suffering from kidney stones, as it contains lot of water in it, so it helps to dissolve the kidney stones fast.
- Grapes juice have an exceptional diuretic value on account of their high contents of water and potassium salt. The value of this fruit in kidney troubles is enhanced by its low albumin and sodium chloride content. It is an excellent cure for kidney stones.
- Lemon juice also helps in dissolving kidney stones, consume lemon juice after a regular interval on daily basis.

IRREGULAR BLEEDING: This is a very common problem seen in women of reproductive age group.

Causes:	Symptoms:
• Imbalance of hormones	• Pain in lower abdomen
• Tension	• Pain in the lumber and hip region.
• Cancer of the uterus	• Weakness and giddiness
	• Breathlessness
	• Palpitation and anaemia

Cure:
* Amla can be eaten daily for controlling bleeding.
* A piece of fresh ginger grounded and boiled in a cup of water. The infusion should be taken thrice daily, after meals along with Honey.

Juice Therapy:

* Grape juice daily can be consumed for restoring regular periods.

* Drink a glass of carrot juice daily for three months. This herbal remedy helps in treating an irregular menstrual cycle.

* Drinking the juice of Bitter Gourd (Karela) daily can also help to regular your periods.

MALARIA: Malaria is a common fever, occurring frequently in tropical regions like India, Africa etc.

Causes:
- Tiny single celled parasite
- Transmitted by the bite of an infected mosquito

Symptoms:
- Severe headache, body ache and pain in the muscles.
- Shivering and high temperature
- Vomiting
- Cycle of fever may come and go

Cure:
- About 15 to 25 ml of Lemon juice should be taken with water.
- Fresh juice extracted from 10 basil leaves (about 10 ml) mixed well with 10 ml of honey should be repeated 4 times a day.

Juice Therapy:
- Papaya leaf juice formula will work for Malaria. In fact whenever there is an infection (bacteria or viral infection) it can be used. Combine it with neem leaves juice; it will become even more potent. Consume 30 ml of neem leaf juice and 15 ml of Papaya leaf juice.
- It is recommended to fast on orange juice and water for some days. The number of days required for fast depends on the severity of the Malarial fever.

MIGRAINE: Migraine is known as sick headache, because nausea and vomiting occasionally accompany the excruciating pain which lasts for as long as three days.

Causes:	Symptoms:
• Severe headache • Disorder of digestion • Under great mental tension	• Blurring of the vision • Feeling of tingling • Numbness • Weakness in an arm or leg

Cure:
- Drinking lemon juice in small quantity frequently brings relief in migraine cases.
- Copious drinking of water can help in migraine.

Juice Therapy:
- Carrot juice, in combination with spinach juice, has been found beneficial in treatment of migraine.

- The juice of grapes is an effective home remedy for a migraine. Drink 50 ml of grape juice in morning for 15 days.

NOSE RUNNING OR BLOCKED (SINUSITIS OR CONGESTION)

It refers to an inflammation of the mucous membrane lining the paranasal sinuses.

Causes:	Symptoms:
• Over-secretion of mucous in the membrane lining the nose, throat and head. • Faulty diet	• Excessive or constant sneezing • Running nose • Blockage of one or both nostrils

Cure:
- Take tulsi leaves along with ginger powder in boiled water.
- Eat pungent herbs like garlic and onion, which tend to break up mucous congestion all through the respiratory tract.
- Drink 50 ml of Amla juice for two weeks.

Juice therapy:
- Consume 20 to 30 ml of fresh Wheatgrass juice daily on empty stomach.

NOSE BLEEDING: Nose bleeding is a common problem that can be treated at home easily. Medically it is known as epitasis.

Causes:	Symptom:
• Cold or flu	• Expelling of blood from the nostril
• Allergies	
• Nasal tumor	
• Nose injury	
• Nasal infection	

Cure:
• Drop lemon juice in the nostrils.
• Use cold compress or an ice pack around the nose.

Juice Therapy :

• Stop nose bleeding by putting a few drops of Pomegranate juice into your nostrils.

• The rich vitamin C in lemon juice helps to heal, repair, build and strengthen the lining of the mucous membranes to prevent nose bleeding.

• Juice of Gooseberry (Amla) is a good remedy to cure nose bleeding.

• Due to cooling properties. Drinking ash Gourd (Petha) juice everyday keeps the body cool and stops nose bleeding.

OBESITY: The term obesity applies when a person has excessive body fats and is at least 20 per cent heavier than he or she should be in proportion to his height and physique.

Causes:	Symptoms:
• Eating too much • Inherited one • Result of hormonal disorder	• Extra accumulated fat on joints of hips, knees, ankles • Coronary thrombosis, heart failure

Cure:

- 1 tsp of honey and fresh juice of half lemon should be mixed well and added to a glass of lukewarm water taken twice or thrice.
- Mix lemon juice with honey and water. Drink it every morning.
- Obesity can also be cured by drinking Aloe Vera juice. It increases the metabolic rate, which will help to burn calories

Juice Therapy:

- Drinking juice of 1 Lemon in a cup of warm water on empty stomach early morning, every day helps in reducing obesity.
- Pineapple juice is also the best to reduce obesity and moreover by having a glass of Pineapple juice we can suppress our appetite too.
- Cantaloupe (Kharbooza) juice is perfect for loosing weight in Obesity.

PILES: It is a thickening and inflammation of veins inside or just outside the rectum.

Causes:	**Symptoms:**
• Persistent constipation and other bowel disorders • Prolonged periods of standing or sitting • Strenuous work • Obesity • General weakness of the tissue of the body • Mental tension • Heredity	• Pain while passing stools • Slight bleeding in the case of internal trouble • Feeling of soreness and irritation after passing a stool • Discomfort around the rectal area.

Cure:

• Grind 1 onion to paste. Mix with curd and eat it once or twice a day for 7 days. Eating raw onion is very good for treating piles.
• For curing Piles, Aloe Vera juice can be consumed; moreover the gel can directly be applied on the infected area.

Juice Therapy:

• Ginger is quite useful in piles treatment. Patients should have half a teaspoon of fresh ginger juice, mixed with one teaspoon of fresh lime juice and 1 tsp of fresh Mint juice along with a tablespoon of Honey. Patients should have it once a day for faster treatment.
• Raw radish juice is a wonderful home remedy for piles. It should be taken two times a day; morning and at night. Drink ¼ cup of radish juice on initial stage and then increase it up to ½ cup.
• Turnip leaves are one of the effective cures for piles. The juice of turnip leaves should be taken twice daily in dosage of 100 ml.

Note: *Avoid Spices and food which is full of chilies. The spicy food is irritant to the intestinal track and causes problems in piles patient. Preserved food, frozen food, canned food, fast food, rich food like pizza's and burgers, noodles and soft drinks should be avoided for treating the piles. Avoid tea and coffee also as they are also bad for piles.*

RHEUMATIC PAIN: Rheumatics refers to pain and swelling of the muscles ,ligaments and tendons or of the joints. It affects men and women ,both young and old.

Causes:	Symptoms:
• Poisoning of the blood and acid wastes	• Intense soreness and pain
• Storage of acidic toxic wastes in the system	• Swollen liver
• By exposure to cold water	• Pain and stiffness

Cure:
• Two or three lemons can be consumed each day.

Juice Therapy
• The juice of raw potato is regarded as excellent remedy for rheumatism. One or two teaspoons of the juice, taken out by pressing mashed raw potatoes, should be taken before meals. This will help to eliminate the toxic condition and relieve rheumatism.
• Consume fresh wheat grass juice up to 20ml to 30ml daily on

RABIES: The bite of a mad dog results in rabies, which can be fatal.

Causes:	Symptoms:
• Virus transmitted to human through the bite of an infected animal	• The patient froths from the mouth
	• He loses his mental balance

Cure:
• Apply fresh onion juice mixed with honey in 2 : 1 ratio on the affected area.

Juice Therapy:
• For rabies wheat grass juice is recommended, as it increases immunity at a very high speed.

SCURVY: It is a deficiency disease that results from insufficient intake of vitamin C.

Causes:	Symptoms:
• Deficiency of vitamin C in the body. • Inadequate intake of fruits and vegetables.	• Breathlessness • Dark purplish spots on skin • Spongy gums often leading to tooth loss • Bleeding gums • Opening of healed scars and separation of bone fractured.

Cure:
• Take 2 to 3 teaspoon of amla juice 2-3 times a day with honey
• Daily intake of lemon juice can also cure scurvy

Juice Therapy:
• In case of scurvy, wheat grass juice is referred as it has high content of chlorophyll and it is also called as green blood, it helps in recovery of scurvy.

WARTS: These are harmless dry growth on the skin

Causes:	Symptoms:
• Caused by virus • Contagious • Spread by touch or through contact	• Small horny lump on the head, face, scalp or knee

Cure:
• Onion pieces when rubbed over the warts cause some irritation. Used over longer periods, warts disappear especially if they are small.

Juice Therapy:
• For curing Warts, squeeze fresh Lemon juice on them three or four times a day. Apply this juice daily, after some days warts will turn black and will separate.

ULCER: Ulcers are wounds that develop on the mucous membranes, when ulcer affects the gastrointestinal tract, they are called peptic ulcers.

Causes:	Symptoms:
• Bacterial infection	• Abdominal pain
• Stress and other psychological factors	• Bloating and abdominal fullness
• Worsened by certain drugs	• Nausea and vomiting
• Hyperactivity due to heavy meals, highly spiced food	• Loss of appetite and weight loss

Cure:

• Raw Honey is an effective treatment for Ulcer. It heals and strengthens the stomach lining.

• Aloe Vera gel works in an amazing way, this gel consumption promotes new cell's formation, so it cures Ulcer at a fast pace.

Juice Therapy:

• 450 ml of Cabbage juice (as a one-time consumption) taken at intervals of few hours everyday can cure ulcers. In most cases pain subsides within five days and healing occurs by the fourteenth day.

• Potato juice when taken alone or in combination with Carrot juice assists in healing intestinal or peptic Ulcer . ½ Potato juice to 1 full glass could be taken 30 minutes before any meal. The initial burning sensation noticed will disappear with subsequent intakes of the Pepper.

BURNING URINATION: While passing urine, some people feel a burning sensation in the urethra.

Causes:	Symptoms:
• Urinary tract infection	• Bleeding in urine
• Venereal diseases	• Fever and stoppage of urination
• Enlarged prostate	• Urine having pus cells
• Stone in urinary bladder	
• Obstruction in urinary passage	

Cure:

• Drinking Barley (Jao) water is good for getting relief in burning urination.

Juice Therapy :

• Take out juice of carrot, celery, and spinach (add a clove of raw garlic). Sip one glass three times daily.

• Lemon juice should be given 2-3 times a day mixed with honey and water.

TUBERCULOSIS: Tuberculosis is a bacterial disease usually affecting the lungs (pulmonary TB). Other parts of the body can also be affected, for example lymph nodes, kidneys, bones, joints, etc.

Symptoms:
- Suffers from constant cough,
- Chronic fever in which the temperature is higher in the evenings
- Lack of appetite,
- Pain in the chest,
- Problem in breathing,
- Excessive mucus of yellowish color

Causes:
- All cases of TB are passed from person to person via droplets.
- Crowded living conditions.
- Alcoholism
- Improper lifestyle

Cure:
- Tuberculosis may also be treated with the Indian Gooseberry (Amla). Mix gooseberry juice with honey and take on a daily basis.
- Consume Bottle Gourd (lauki) juice, as it is one of the best vegetables for treating Tuberculosis.

Juice Therapy:
- Having Apples juice is beneficial for patients of' tuberculosis. Daily consumption of 200 ml apple juice cures Tuberculosis.
- Grape juice in case of tuberculosis helps in getting relief from tuberculosis.
- Taking Carrot juice is helpful. It contains nutrients in a balanced form and helping in recovering Tuberculosis at a high speed.

LOW BLOOD PRESSURE: It is also known as Hypotension, it occurs when blood pressure during and after each heartbeat is much lower than usual. This means the heart, brain, and other parts of the body do not get enough blood.

Symptoms:	Causes:
• Blurry vision	• Use of excessive painkillers
• Feel dizziness	• Dehydration
• Sleepiness all the day	• Heart attack
• Feel weakness	• Alcohol

Cure:·

• Crush 10-15 holy Basil leaves (Tulsi) and strain through a clean muslin cloth. Mix with 1 tsp Honey. Have it the first thing in the morning.

• The best and the most effective home remedy for treating low blood pressure would be to consume lots of water. This is because Dehydration reduces blood volume and leads to a drop in the blood pressure.

Juice Therapy:·

• Consume wheat grass juice up tp 20 to 25 ml in early morning as it will regulate hormonal level.

• Beetroot juice is beneficial for those suffering from low blood pressure. So, have a cup of raw Beetroot juice two times a day.

DENGUE: Dengue fever (also known as break bone fever), is an infectious tropical disease caused by the dengue virus.

Symptoms:	Causes:
• High fever, up to 105 F • Severe headache, backache or both • Pain behind your eyes • Severe joint and muscle pain • Nausea and vomiting	• Blood vessel fluid (Plasma) leakage • Heavy bleeding • A sudden drop in blood pressure

Cure:·

• To lower the fever you should also make sure that the patient drinks a lot of water so that the water balance and blood pressure are under control.

• Prepare some tea using half a teaspoon of fenugreek seeds. Boil it till the water quantity is reduced to half. Drink this tea three times a day. This remedy is very useful in the treatment for dengue fever.

Juice Therapy:·

• 20ml of raw papaya leaf juice, taken twice a day can help dengue patients increase their platelet count and therefore overcome the fever.

• Orange juice is a good source for fighting fevers. It promotes antibodies for speedy recovery and provides energy and vitamins.

• Consume wheat grass juice up to 20 to 25 ml in early morning as it will increase immunity to fight.

CHICKEN POX: Chicken pox is one of the classic childhood diseases. A child or adult with chicken pox may develop hundreds of itchy, fluid-filled blisters that burst and form crusts. Chicken pox is caused by a virus.

Symptoms:	Causes:
• A fever, headache, tummy ache, or loss of appetite for a day or two • Blisters often appear first on the face, trunk, or scalp • Then the blisters become cloudy and then scab.	• From touching the fluids from a chickenpox blister. • Weak immune system • Spread very easily from one to other. • Through an illness or medicines such as chemotherapy and steroids.

Cure:
- In a lukewarm bath, throw in a handful of neem leaves and it will help speed up recovery of chickenpox and relieve itchiness.
- Smear the skin with organic honey and let it absorb into the skin. This will help quickly heal chicken pox.

Juice Therapy:
- To begin with, the patient should be put on a juice diet for a few days. He should be given plenty of raw fruit and vegetable juices. Lemon juice is considered to be especially beneficial.
- The raw Bitter Ggourd juice gives an instant complete relief.

HIGH BLOOD PRESSURE: Blood pressure is the force of blood pushing against blood vessel walls. The heart pumps blood into the arteries (blood vessels), which carry the blood throughout the body. High blood pressure, also called hypertension.

Symptoms:	**Causes:**
• Headache,	• Smoking
• Dizziness,	• Being overweight or obese
• Blurred vision,	• Lack of physical activity
• Nausea and vomiting, and	• Too much salt in the diet
• Chest pain and shortness of breath	• Stress

Cure:
- Mix 1 tsp honey with 1 tsp Ginger juice and 1 tsp cumin powder. Have twice a day.
- A clove of Garlic is highly recommended for high blood pressure. Chew one clove of garlic first thing every morning and wash it down with water. The Garlic can also be coarsely pound and swallowed with water.

Juice Therapy:
- Celery juice has a mild diuretic effect, similar to many drugs that are prescribed for high blood pressure.
- Consume Watermelon juice in order to regulate high blood pressure.

CHAPTER -SIXTEEN

SUPER SPECIALTY HOME HOSPITAL (CLEANSING)STEP -6

Imagine you are eating the best food on the planet, but in a dirty utensil. It will be of little or no use, eating such a food 'garnished with microbes. So, first step towards eating a nutritious food is to get a clean container free of harmful viruses and bacterias.

Similarly body cleansing, is just as important-and even necessary before the vital nutrients can be made available to your cells. By cleansing I mean the removal of metabolic wastes and excess accumulations of foreign matter such as protein, mucous, liquid, fat, calcium, and other minerals; metals like mercury, lead, cadmium, arsenic, aluminum; chemical residues from food additives, drugs, food sprays, and air pollution; radiations from X-rays, and so on.

Modern living has made it difficult for the eliminative organs the colon, skin, kidneys, liver, and lungs to function normally. Not only do they have to perform their normal cleansing functions but they have to combat with a diet composed of high acids. Processed food like burgers, pizzas, chips, french fries, white flour, cereals, refined sugar, milk and animal food have thousands of chemicals and additives in them. Our digestive system simply wasn't set up to perfectly separate the nutrition from the chemicals, and some potentially harmful residues may be retained by the body.

The blood in our veins carries waste to the organs of elimination. If these organs are functioning poorly, because they are clogged with debris, they cannot remove all the waste from the blood. Unable to carry more toxins in solution, the blood compels the ten trillion body cells to accumulate waste to their capacity. It is similar to what occurred in New Delhi, during the garbage collector's strike several years ago. The dumps were closed, refusing to accept any more garbage; and the sanitation collectors wouldn't pick up the trash from home. Buildings overflowed with garbage and then flooded the streets. Soon the city was filled with trash.

To clean up the mess, it was necessary to open the dumps (organs) to allow the men and trucks to empty the trash, they removed from the cans (cells). Before true health or reversal of symptoms can occur, waste products must be cleared from the cells, blood, and organs of the body. Sooner this is accomplished, the sooner body will repair itself.

During the process of cleansing the colon, liver, lungs, kidneys, and skin; vital nutrients in the diet reach the cells and stimulate an increased metabolic rate. This speeds the elimination of waste products from the cells into the bloodstream, which in turn places a greater burden on the major eliminative organs.

I suggest you a cleansing regime for 10 days. During this time you will notice, on some days your energy level is super high while you experience a big 'low' on the other days. But dear friends, this is quite natural rather these fluctuations are a good indicator of the cycles of cleansing your body is passing through. As debris is released and removed from your system, your energy level surges up but as soon as your blood and organs of elimination become congested with debris brought from other organs, you feel tired again.

To cure these fluctuations, try to eat three meals daily.

Include only the following foods in your meals every day:

➢   5-7 servings of fresh fruits

➢   2 to 3 large bowls green salads

➢   2 cups of sprouts

➤ One glass of green drink (vegetables)

➤ 50 ml of Wheatgrass juice, the first thing in the morning.

➤ 8 to 10 glasses of water (water kept in copper jug overnight).

➤ Be sure to take plenty of rest and do some exercise each day preferably walking or stretching for 1 hour.

➤ Also perform the non dietary cleansing techniques as given below in following pages.......

CLEANSING THE COLON

The colon is the body's main avenue for physical elimination of waste. The modern sedentary lifestyle, characterized by a diet high in animal's fat, proteins, artificial and refined foods, has made the colon resemble a sewer system. Like a cesspool, it may breed millions of harmful bacterias and emit foul and embarrassing gasses.

Here is quick picture to give you a visual idea.

This putrefaction and decay that stagnates in the colon eventually seeps through the walls and enters the blood stream. Circulating throughout the blood stream these poisons eventually hit every organ in the body;

➤ Causes brain and nervous system damage that make us depressed and irritable.

➤ Causes the heart to weaken.

➤ Causes the liver and gallbladder to become so clogged that they cannot function properly (which in turn creates the bloating sensation after eating).

➤ Causes the skin to look sallow and unhealthy.

These things mentioned above will make you look and feel older, your joints get stiffed and painful, your eyes become dull and your brain sluggish as your body prematurely ages from the burden of too much accumulated acidic waste.

BEST WAY TO CLEAN THE COLON-ENEMA

Steps of Enema:

1. Do not consume anything at night before going for enema next morning.

2. Take an Enema bag.

3. Take a glass of clean water and add ½ glass of wheat grass juice.

4. Fill your enema bag with clean water dissolved with Wheatgrass juice and hang it as high as possible somewhere in the bathroom. Just make sure that the tip extends near enough to reach you.

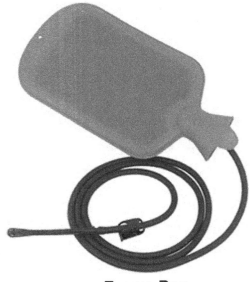

Enema Bag

5. Fold a towel few times and place it on the bathroom floor under your knees, if you have a hard bathroom floor.

6. Lubricate the tip of enema bag with the oil and put a little on the anus too, if required.

7. Release the plastic clamp over the toilet or sink until you see water flowing. This will push out whatever air is left in the tube.

8. Squat down on knees and bend forward. Make sure your knees are spread apart so that they are not applying pressure on the abdominal region.

9. Slowly insert the tip of enema bag into the rectum and release the plastic clamp for the water to flow in.

10. As the water flows in take deep breaths pushing the stomach out

after each inhale. This will release even more pressure on the abdomen.

11. If you start feeling uncomfortable just push the clamp, so that the water stops flowing and get up to let it out in the toilet. Take a few deep breaths and when the irritation has stopped then release the clamp again for more water to enter. Continue doing this until you can retain the whole bag of water.

ADVANCED COLON CLEANSING

After 3 to 4 days of Enema you can now prepare yourself for much advanced colon cleansing i.e.

WHEATGRASS IMPLANT

To use, 'Wheatgrass juice implants' as a purge, simply fill a sterilized infant enema syringe with 30 ml of fresh juice and insert it into the rectum. A couple of minutes later, the bowels will move hurriedly. Try another 30 ml implant and also let it out, if you feel the urge to pass it out. The second attempt will probably carry more faecal matter with it. A third implant, 60 ml will usually be retained with ease. Hold it in until you feel the urge to eliminate, generally about twenty minutes later. There is no danger of reabsorbing toxins, if you have purged the colon first with other implants or enemas. You may even be surprised to find that all the juice has been totally absorbed inside you.

To perform the implant after you have cleansed the colon, simply lean towards one side while on the toilet seat and use an infant Enema syringe to squeeze the juice into the rectum. Make sure that all the equipment you use is sterile. 60 ml of juice can be comfortably retained in the colon.

Try to hold the juice fifteen minutes to an hour before expelling it.

The quantity of wheat grass juice can be taken between 30 ml to 60 ml depending upon person to person.

CLEANSING THE LIVER

Since liver is the major organ of detoxification, it determines the health of the other organs and the blood. The liver is a processing plant and storage place for metabolic wastes and pollutants, as well as many nutrients. The food of the modern diet, especially meats, fried foods, refined oils, and foods with chemical additives weaken the liver. Alcohol, tobacco and environmental pollutants add extra duties to the already known 260 functions of the liver.

To regain health and energy, the liver and gall bladder must be cleansed and kept free flowing. To achieve it, the best way is to drink 60 ml of wheat grass juice for 3 to 4 weeks early in the morning with empty stomach. It contains an abundance of magnesium, enzymes, chlorophyll, protein and full range of vitamins and minerals.

½ lemon juice and 2 table spoon of honey added to a glass of Luke warm water can work as an excellent cleansing agent and known for its antiseptic action. Drink it 3 to 4 times a day for 4 weeks.

CLEANSING THE LUNGS

Without food we can live for months and without liquids we can survive for days, but breath is life. Without breathing, we can live just for a few minutes. Perhaps this is the reason why, almost all ancient cosmologies and religions made so many references to the breath. Breathing is our link with the atmosphere, the ocean, the trees and the plants, whose leaves convert human carbon dioxide waste into a fresh supply of oxygen. When our lungs are congested with mucous and burdened by excessive carbon waste products, our vital lung's capacity is reduced and we no longer have sufficient amounts of oxygen to burn up bodily wastes.

BREATHING EXERCISES

The body's supply of oxygen is largely responsible for the oxidation or burning up of toxins. Most adults use only one quarter of their lung capacity, when breathing normally. However, during breathing exercises, at least three-quarters of this capacity is put to use, adding a tremendous amount of oxygen to the blood. In fact, if you are new to deep breathing, the release of added oxygen into the blood could leave you feeling lightheaded.

Deep breathing should begin in the stomach, pushing the diaphragm down and out. Make sure you are sitting comfortably, with the spine erect and the entire body relaxed. Now let the inhaled air fill the middle and upper regions of the lungs. You will notice the abdomen automatically contracting and the shoulders going back as you fill the upper chest. Now, without holding your breath, release the air slowly, in reverse order, contracting the chest first and then the abdomen. If you feel lightheaded and dizzy, stop. Otherwise, repeat this exercise atleast fifteen times. (Take rest for five minutes between the breaths).

Yet another way to clean the lungs is by drinking Wheatgrass juice as its chemical make up is similar to the red blood cells, chlorophyll of the Wheatgrass increases the red blood cell count in the body enabling the blood to carry more oxygen and remove more acidic waste.

CLEANSING THE KIDNEYS

Every day, four thousand quarts of blood flows through your kidneys, where it is cleansed of metabolic waste, urea, uric acid, excess water and other metabolic waste products are eliminated and the acid-alkaline balance of the blood is maintained by the kidneys. Without their vital cleansing assistance, you would die of autointoxication in a few hours. Body temperature is also regulated by the kidneys. Considered "the seat of life" by Oriental doctors, the kidneys are believed by many people to be closely linked with reproductive functions and willpower. They are also responsible for eliminating drugs, pollutants, and bacterial waste from the body.

The kidneys are perhaps the most stressed of all organs in modern people. With several thousand additives and drugs finding their way into our food and water, the kidneys have an extra full time job. Inside each kidney, millions of vitally important little filters called nephrons are damaged by the acidic toxins. Unfortunately, many people don't experience symptoms of kidney damage until 90 percent of the function is lost, and at this stage the damage is life threatening.

The first step in healing the kidneys is to avoid all refined, processed foods, salt, meat, coffee, tea, alcohol, tobacco, and tap water.

The course of therapy we recommend for strengthening and cleansing the kidneys is safe and effective. The active elements in this procedure are listed below.

➤ Green drinks (green vegetables)

➤ Wheatgrass juice acts as a diuretic and stimulant for increased kidney filtration of waste. Its chlorophyll content helps rebuild the blood and relieves the kidneys of their burden.

CHAPTER -SEVENTEEN

GUIDED IMAGINARY METHOD
STEP -7

To understand the mechanism of mind-body model of recovery take this example. Imagine that you are having a stock of following things and resources:-

1. Brick
2. Cement
3. Labour force
4. Mud and Clay
5. Rock
6. Concrete
7. Glass

And finally an appropriate land and you are the architect of building that is being made out of it and now depends solely on the architect that is – you. Regarding what to do with the available resources. The same resource may be converted into a school or into a temple if you like, or into a hospital or a pollution producing industrial building.

The resources and the material remains the same, what makes the difference is the instruction of the architect i.e. you.

Similar is the case with the body. Your body is the collection of all the required material to build a beautiful life, but the architect of the body is your mind. Remember, what we think with full faith and belief about our body's physical well being gets translated into the equivalent physical being. By repeated mental focusing about the well being of a particular organ, the brain creates a specific neural network resulting in the physical change in the well being of the organ being imagined. This concept in neuroscience is called Hebbian Learning. This mind-body principle can be used to get recovery from all kind of diseases.

Figure given below summarizes how mind and body can interact to create health. The explanation starts again in the psychological realm.

Psychological Intervention

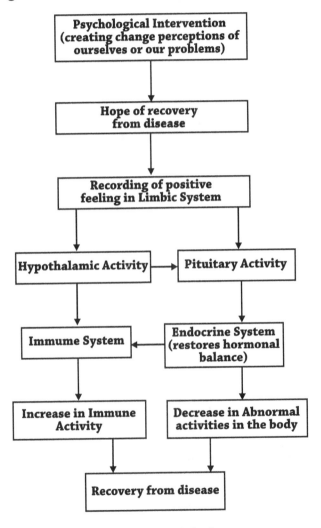

A Mind / Body Model of Recovery

The first step towards the recovery is to assist yourself in strengthening your belief in the effectiveness of Wheatgrass therapy and the potency of your body's defenses. Then you can learn to cope more effectively with the stresses in your life. It is particularly important that there can be a change either in your perceptions of yourself so you believe you can solve whatever life problems you faced before the onset of the disease or in your perception of your problems so that you believe you can cope with yourself more effectively.

Hope of Recovery from Disease
The results of your beliefs in your opportunities for recovery, coupled with your "redecision" about the problems you face, are an approach to life that includes hope and anticipation.

↓

Recovery of Positive Feeling
Renewed feelings of hope and anticipation are recorded in the limbic system.

↓

Hypothalamic Activity
Once these feelings are recorded in the limbic system, messages are sent to the hypothalamus reflecting the altered emotional state that includes an increased will to live. The hypothalamus then sends messages to the pituitary gland that reflect the altered emotional state.

↓

Immune System
The hypothalamus in turn reverses the suppression of the immune system, so that the body's defenses once again mobilize, against abnormal activities in the body.

↓

↓

Pituitary Activity/Endocrine System

The pituitary gland (which is part of the endocrine system), receiving messages from the hypothalamus, sends messages to the rest of the endocrine system, restoring the body's hormonal balance.

↓

Decrease in Abnormal Activities in the Body

With the hormonal balance restored, the body will discontinue abnormal activities in the body and body starts revitalizing its defense system to cope with the illness.

Step by step methods of using mind power to guide your body to a super recovery from a disease.

You may tape-record the following steps as it may prove helpful to you in the process of doing the following mental exercise. It should take 10 to 15 minutes to complete the entire process and you should practice it 3 times a day specially immediately after having Wheatgrass shot (we will understand more about wheat grass therapy in the subsequent chapters) and also just before going to the bed at night.

1. Go to a quiet room with soft green lighting. Shut the door, sit in a comfortable chair, feet flat on the floor, eyes closed.

2. Become aware of your breathing.

3. Take in a few deep breaths, and as you let out each breath, mentally say the word, "relax."

4. Concentrate on your face and feel if any tension in the muscles of your face and around your eyes. Make a mental picture of this tension it might be a rope tied in a knot or a clenched fist and then mentally picture it relaxing and becoming loose, like a limp rubber band.

5. Experience the muscles of your face and eyes getting relaxed. As they relax, feel a wave of relaxation spreading through your body.

6. Tense the muscles of your face and around your eyes, squeezing tightly, then relax them and feel the relaxation spreading through your body.

7. More slowly down your body-jaw, neck, shoulders, back, upper and lower arms, hands, chest, abdomen, thighs, calves, ankles, feet-until every part of your body is more relaxed. For each part of the body mentally picture the tension, and then picture the tension melting away, allowing relaxation.

8. Now picture yourself in pleasant, natural surroundings wherever you fee comfortable. Mentally fill in the details of color, sound, and texture.

9. Continue to picture yourself in a very relaxed state in this natural place for two to three minutes.

10. Create a mental picture of any ailment or pain that you have now, visualizing it in a form that makes sense to you.

11. As you are inhaling deep, visualize a shower of green light (similar to wheat grass juice) entering in your body through your mouth and falling on the diseased organ or the body parts with pain, with a great impact.

12. Imagine the diseased organ getting heated due to the power of green light. Also picture your body's natural defense and natural process eliminating the source of the ailment or pain.

13. Imagine yourself healthy and free of the ailment or pain.

14. See yourself proceeding successfully towards meeting your goal in life.

15. Give yourself mental pat on the back for participating in your recovery. See yourself doing this relaxation mental imaginary exercise, staying awake and alert as you do it.

16. Let the muscles in your eyelids lighten up, become ready to open your eyes, and become aware of the room.

17. Now let your eyes open and you are ready to resume your usual routine activities.

Now, allow me to give you some curing techniques for a few 'stubborn' and 'common' diseases......

This can be done anywhere, anytime but I will suggest you to follow the Super Specialty Master Plan in chapter 15. But make it a point not to miss it.

For curing any disease step 1- 9 and 12 - 17 will be the same. The only deviation will be from step 10 to step11. I shall be discussing only these for specific diseases in following pages.

CAD (Coronary Heart Disease)
Follow instructions till 9.

Step 10: Now, take a few deep breaths, imagine yourself breathing bright, green, intense light, coming from universe. Visualize that the light is entering through your nostrils to your lungs and then spreading through your entire body. You feel a 'glow' in your body.

Step 11: Develop an image of rays passing through the blocked arteries. Initially they will not be able to pass....because of blockage. Now imagine them as laser grinder blades moving in circles. Light moving fast..... very fast......try to hear that cracking... and crushing sound inside your body and produce the same sound from your mouth slowly.... Krrrr..... krrrrrrr...... feel the grinding of the blocks in arteries.

Step 12: Experience the blocked plaques melting down and fresh blood gustily flowing through arteries. Imagine the blocks getting reduced, flow of blood becoming normal... Feel a sense of warmth, freshness and rejuvination.

HYPHERTENSION

This will not only prevent hypertension but also treat and cure the one you have.

Follow the instructions from step 1- 9.

Step 10: Make a mental picture of the heart beating blood flowing through the narrow periphery of limbs. It is causing strain on heart and arteries. The pressure inside heart and arteries is increasing.

Step 11: Imagine that you are inhaling fresh air and bright and warm green light. Your lungs are filled with this air and light. It is spreading over your body and all the organs become shiny and bright.

Step 12: The light you are inhaling is going through the narrow segments causing relaxation and dilation. The pressure and strain is gradually decreasing and heart is beating normally without strain. Feel the lowering of blood pressure.

Feel relaxed and free from tension.

Repeat the process 3-4 times.

You will see your headache reducing and disappearing....the strain from your head has vanished...

SLEEP DISORDERS

By this technique I ensure you good sleep....even in a rocking party.

Step 10: Imagine yourself to be on a peaceful beach, or a calm sea or in a beautiful garden. You can imagine a beautiful, natural place of your choice.

Step 11: Make a mental picture of yourself walking on the selected spot. Increase the speed.....feel the grass/sand.....walk fast, even faster, now start 'jogging' feel the touch of ground. You are sweating and feeling tired after the jog. Feel the strain on muscles and fatigue in your legs.

Step 12: Slow down the speed and walk normally... stop walking and stand still. Now lay comfortable on ground, body relaxing. Feel the grass/sand and the touch of ground.

Feel someone massaging you. Feel the comfort in limbs. Breathe the stroke of fresh air.....

Are you sleepy....your eyes are drooping and you gradually fall asleep.

WOUND HEALING

Yes, don't be surprised... you can heal your wounds too.....

Step 10: Imagine a ray of bright green light coming from universe and falling upon your wound. See your wound is bathing in the bright green light and is being soothed.

Step 11: The wound slowly being filled with red tissue; the light is now causing a mild irritation... Feel the itch...ohhhh...

Step 12 : Gradually the wound is filled with normal tissue. Starting from periphery towards the centre. The skin gaps are reducing. Skin over the wound thickens. It is now just like before. Feel that there is no pain and feeling left.

Your wound is healed.....

IRRITABLE BOWEL SYNDROME

Step 10: Visualize your intestines....

Step 11: Imagine yourself in tense position.....angry. Shouting at someone, who is not obeying you. See yourself getting abdominal pain, slight discomfort in the abdomen... Feel the pain.

Step 12: See yourself lying down at your favorite place, feel the freshness of air. Imagine the green light falling on your abdomen. Gradually the light is making your intestines recoil fast. It is having a soothing and calming effect on your brain and abdomen. Your intestines are reducing their movement and moving at a normal pace feel the gut. Your intestines are relaxing. The gas in the intestine is slowly getting absorbed and expelled out.

GLAUCOMA

You must have seen people getting miraculously healed at religious places... yes this is true.... they are healed by their mind power...the inner strength. Religious places offer a motivation to excite the mind power to peak.

Step 10: Imagine your eyes as two spheres....each eye having six green balls representing obstructions. Visualize the green light rays falling on your both eyes. See that the rays are gradually hitting the balls causing abstraction.(play billiards). These are milling and falling down, one by one ...

Step 11: Now your eyes are free from the blocks. This happens in both the eyeballs, one by one.

Step 12: Feel the increased flow of 'aqueous humor' in your eyes. Feel relaxed, free of tension and headache.

Your eye balls are now completely free from strain...

BACKACHE

It is a very common ailment. It is a gift of modern lifestyle.

Step 10: Make a mental picture of your spine.

Step 11: Imagine, your spine is rigid and stiff.

Visualize someone massaging your spine. up... and... down, feel the pressure. Feel the pressure of aching muscles.

Step 12: Imagine a ray of green light falling on your spine and is slowly moving downward. It is relaxing your muscles.... ligaments....joints... gradually... feel the disappearance of rigidity...feel the relaxation. Repeat at least six times.

CONSTIPATION

Step 10: Imagine a large colon loaded with faeces. Do deep abdominal breathing at least six times.

Step 11: See a ray of green light falling on your colon. Feel the abdominal muscles contracting and relaxing, and putting pressure on your colon.

Step 12: Visualize the faeces in your rectum gradually moving lower. Feel the pressure and egest...

MIGRAINE

Imagine your aching head....

Step 10: Sit comfortably ...... take 5-6 deep abdominal breaths... recall a picture of any loved one. (your mother, wife, daughter, son...)

Step 11: Visualize a green ray of light falling on your forehead. See the nerves calming down and the face of your loved one soothing your head.

Step 12: Feel yourself to be relaxing and de-stressing, and your migraine has gone...

Note : *It is advised to follow the above technique at least for 21 days, 3 times a day for a tangible result.*

NOTHING IS IMPOSSIBLE FOR A WILLING HEART

CHAPTER -EIGHTEEN

SUPER SPECIALTY MASTER PLAN (S²MP) STEP -8

When we talk of diet plan, we talk mostly of what to eat. But that's always confusing. Let's start with something to avoid. Things 'not to be eaten'.

The following maxim has the potential to make your life disease free and lend you a long and healthy life.

"If it is man made – don't eat".

Remember anything which is packed and found on the shelf having a shelf life, is poisonous for the body. You may call it a dead food. It includes not only chips, cold drinks, sauces, packed breads, ice- creams and curd but also all kinds of conventional medicines found in the chemist store. Let's understand the difference between the live and the dead food.

Living food v/s Dead food

This is where you should put your concentration the most; the stuff you put into your body, named as 'food' and that you chew and swallow it with great charm but think, if your body is equally charmed too.

We need to make a big differentiation within foods.

➢ Living Food- Any food that is in its their natural state, unadulterated by man, e.g. fruits, sprouted grains, raw honey, soaked nuts, and vegetables.

➢ Dead Food – Any food that has been over cooked, pasteurized, micro waved, homogenized, processed, or adulterated e.g. burger, chips, noodles, canned food, bakery items, bread, condensed milk etc.

Out of the trillions of different species on this planet, from the microscopic bugs in the dirt, to the birds in the air, to the depths of the ocean, we humans are the only ones who cook and mix our foods. And don't think even for a second that it's supposedly because we have intelligence. But in fact, it is quite the opposite. We have been actually destroying our nature food.

There are several things that happen to food when it is being cooked. Every time you heat a piece of food over $118°$ F for 3 minutes, you destroy 100% of the enzymes, almost all the vitamins and minerals. Over heating of fats and proteins denatures the chemical structures, creating indigestible carcinogens. These indigestible wastes are very harsh for the body. Under high heat, natural sugar become caramelized and the natural fibers of food are broken down into useless substances, which in turn, make food stay longer in digestive tract.

All living foods are composed of living cells. When you eat this living food the life force is transferred to your cells adding life force to your body. When food is cooked and processed you do receive calories and sometimes a small amount of nutrients but NO 'life force'. So, it is quite ostensible that a food that contains living cells is definitely superior.

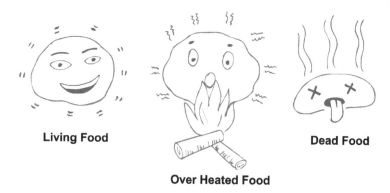

Living Food　　　　　**Dead Food**

Over Heated Food

This should be fairly easy to comprehend. What happens when you put anything on fire?

It breaks down and is destroyed.

So what happens when this damaged (or burnt) food enter the body!

Heating sugar, fat, and protein makes them inorganic matter. These inorganic elements enter the blood stream and circulate through your body settling in the arteries, veins and deaden the nerves. These are the accumulations that cause thousands of different diseases such as arthritis, heart disease, colon cancer, etc....

Eventually the body looses its flexibility, our nerves begin to lose the power of conveying messages, our spinal cord becomes hardened, and tissues throughout the body contract and our bodies become prematurely old.

The constant fight against the toxic effects of processed and over cooked foods unnecessarily exhausts the body's strength and vitality, thus causing disease and shortening of life.

THE PURPOSE OF FIBER

The fibers of natural food act as a broom inside our intestines, which help to grab hold of waste matter and pass it through the intestines. Over cooking destroys this fiber making it too soft.

Fibrous material should be somewhat rough and tough and hence, the other popular name for fiber "roughage." Food is pushed through the body by muscles and hair like structures on the inner walls of the intestines. This is called peristaltic action. The intestine needs this type of "roughage" so that it has something more solid to grab a hold of and push through your internal pipes. Without this fiber the intestines have nothing to work against. This makes it hard to pass the waste material through the intestines. When waste material is not quickly passed, it ferments and begins to putrefy in the intestinal tract. These waste materials then start to accumulate and line the walls of the large and small intestines. In due course they accumulate so much garbage and debris that they become clogged.

On the next page is a simple drawing to give you a better mental picture of waste material built up on the walls of the colon and how fiber acts as a broom to help grab it and sweep it away.

Ninety percent of the vitamins and minerals of food are absorbed through the walls of the small intestine. When they are lined with putrefactive matter, only minuscule amounts of nutrients are absorbed. Also, this waste matter slowly leaks through the walls of the intestines and circulated back into the blood stream creating what is called autointoxication (basically the body poisoning itself). Sometimes they

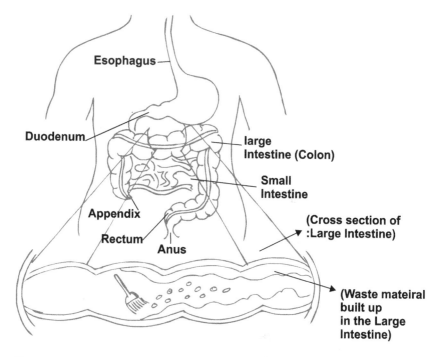

Esophagus

Duodenum

large
Intestine (Colon)

Small
Intestine

Appendix

(Cross section of
:Large Intestine)

Rectum

Anus

(Waste mateiral
built up
in the Large
Intestine)

**(The Broom Represents Fiber Grabbing And Sweeping Old Waste Material
Through The Colon)**

become so clogged that nothing passes through, creating serious problems such as constipation and much more.

Have you ever felt hunger pangs shortly after you have just eaten!

Many over cooked and processed foods are devoid of proper nutrients and now your body cries out to eat again so that it is supplied with the proper nutrients.

Over cooked food has less nutrition so now you will have the tendency to eat more and more for your appetite to be satisfied. And of course when you eat more cooked food you will get fatter and unhealthy much easily.

So what are the benefits we receive when we eat living foods!

1. Living foods are digested and pass through the body very easily. They contain their own enzymes. These enzymes help to break the food down in your stomach reducing large amount of burden from your body to handle this process.

2. Living foods do not leave you with tired feeling, most of the people experience after eating a cooked meal.

3. Your mind will be clearer. You will be much more alert, think sharper and be more logical. If you are a student studying for a test or one who has to be mentally alert at work, you will notice a big difference after eating living food.

4. The nutrients of these foods will be fully absorbed by the body, which will leave you more satisfied. Then you will have the tendency to eat less and more contented.

5. These foods will clean the body. After a few months on living foods halitosis and body odor will be eliminated. You won't even need deodorant, saving you tons of money over the years.

6. Your eyes will become clearer and colour in your eyes brighter.

7. Your skin will start to glow and become very smooth, which will make you look much younger.

8. You will have way more energy and need less sleep. But you will have to have much more restful sleep.

After a short time a peaceful wave will flow through your body and your nerves will be much calmer. You will worry a lot less about the crazy little things that we tend to get so wrapped up in.

It is truly an amazing experience when the body is cleansed on living foods. You will start to see life in a new way that you never had before.

The Real Secret Behind Living Food is Enzyme

Enzymes are the body's labor force. They are the construction and demolition teams that work twenty four hours a day to build, repair, and maintain balance in the body.

The only reason you are alive is because of thousands of enzymes. They are the energy force or "metabolites" of the body. Without them we would be a lifeless glop of proteins, vitamins, minerals, and water.

They perform every function in the body. Every breath you take, every thought you think or sentence you read is the result of thousands of complex enzyme system and their functions operating simultaneously.

Again, living foods contain their own enzymes, which help to break themselves down in your digestive tract for assimilation and evacuation. These enzymes are the reason why fruit ripens or "breaks down". As you can see when a banana turns from green to yellow to brown, this is the movement of enzymes.

It's the same reason papayas get sweeter, enzymes are performing their natural job of breaking these foods down into simpler substances so that the body can use them.

This you do not find in processed foods at the grocery stores. That is why they stay the same no matter what. They are basically a lifeless pile of chemicals manufactured into a certain form. Being the lifeless structure, these food sit in the departmental store shelves for months. This way, who ever sells them, can make more money, because they don't have to throw them away so quickly.

LOSING ENERGY FROM PROCESSED FOODS

When we eat processed and cooked foods, which are devoid of enzymes, there is an internal alarm that goes off inside the stomach. This alarm calls on our own body's enzymes to come and help break down these lifeless substances because the food's enzymes have been destroyed through heat and processing.

This is why most people loose energy and concentration after eating cooked meals. The body's own enzymes that were performing other functions such as thinking, muscle reparation, etc.... now have to stop what they are doing and help aid in the digestion process. This leaves us with that tired feeling most of us can relate after eating a heavily cooked meal especially after that big New Year dinner.

The more you use them up the shorter your life will be. When we eat cooked food or food processed with chemicals, drink alcohol, use drugs and stimulants, it uses a tremendous supply of our own limited amount of enzymes to deal with and rid the body of these things.

Medical research has shown that allergies, skin disorders, heart diseases, obesity, certain types of cancer, and ageing are all seen in people with enzyme deficiencies.

So if you want to loose fat, calcium deposits in joints, cholesterol in your arteries, or break down cancerous tumors, it is enzymes who will perform these functions. We must learn to eat living foods that contain their own enzymes so that our body's enzymes can take care of other tasks instead of working on digestion.

The same applies when we want to build our muscles, have strong teeth, better eyesight, repair wounds, etc... we must keep our body's enzymes free from having to do so much digestion. Just to add high – quality proteins and vitamins and minerals will not do. We need the metabolic process of living enzymes to build muscles, new blood, bones, nerves, and healthy tissues.

So bottom line, we truly need living food if we really want to be alive. Not just live, but be alive!

Awareness of Fruits: The best food for human body is the fruit. It is created by the nature in such a way that it is digested in body within 30 to

40 minutes. Whereas, a continental lunch or dinner meal, takes around 2 to 4 hours for digestion. So it should be the first thing to be eaten in the morning to replete the nutrients. We must not choke our body with the loads of cooked and processed food in the morning, and putting an undue, heavy burden on the body. This results in a fatigue syndrome, at the start of the day. Rather we need a quick bust of energy in the morning so as to kick start the day. Fruits are the best choice. Fruits are loaded with enzymes, vitamins, minerals, lot of fibers and oxygen. Remember not to mix fruit with any other kind of food.

After the awareness about the mind, body, food, truths about medicine and the mechanism of the disease, its time to create a Super Specialty Master Plan (S^2MP) which can not only help us to reverse all kinds of diseases and restore a normal health but also increase the longevity and vitality of the life. This Super Specialty Master Plan is inspired by the life style of two of the healthiest culture of the earth i.e. the Vilcabambas of Ecuador and the Hunzas of the Himalayas.

Here is a land where people do not have common diseases like us, such as heart ailments, cancer, arthritis, high blood pressure, diabetes, tuberculosis, hay fever, asthma, liver trouble, gall bladder trouble, constipation or many other ailments that plague the rest of the world. Moreover, there are no hospitals, no insane asylums, no drug stores, no saloons, no tobacco stores, no police, no jails, no crimes, no murders, and no beggars.

These people are commonly found living to be 100,110,120 and occasionally as much as 140 years of age.

Super Specialty Master Plan

For next 31 days to reverse any disease and reclaim health.

Step 1 : 10 days of cleansing as discussed in the previous chapter.

Step 2: Follow the remedy as given in the applications section for on average 10 days (depending on the severity of the disease) during the cleansing period.

Step 3: After the first 10 days of the cleansing and the applications period, follow the final Super Specialty Master Plan for next 31 days.

Super Specialty Master Plan (S^{2}MP)

5.00 am : Wheat grass juice (50 to 100 ml)

5:15 am : 15 minutes of mental imagery to treat the specific disease (as given is chapter 14).

6:00 am to 11:00 am: Lots of fresh fruit diet of your choice.

1:00 pm: Low cooked simple vegetarian meal of your choice. This should be the heaviest meal of the day, as it is scientifically proven that around 1:00 pm body's capacity to digest and assimilate food is the highest.

Around 4:00 pm: Wheat grass juice (50 ml to 100 ml)

Between 6.00 to 7.00 pm: Lots of fresh fruits.

Around 8.00 pm: Lots of lightly boiled vegetables.

Around 10.00 pm: 15 minutes of mental imagery to treat the specific disease.

Around 10:15 pm: Going for a good night sleep.

General Instructions:

1. Drink around 8 to 10 glasses of water from copper jug (to be stored for 24 hrs before consumption) as it has various curative properties including relieving pain, healing wound and maintaining digestive health. Avoid drinking water just before the main meal (at least ½ hr before/ 1 hr after the main meal).

2. Keep some time for recreation/hobby or just watch some funny videos.

3. Spend one hour for any kind of exercise including walking, running, stretching or any physical sports. The best time to do it is before the sunrise or the sunset.

4. Avoid combining various kinds of food. Primitive man never used to collect various kinds of food at one place then mixing it together before eating. Our stomach is designed to handle one kind of food at a time. Human beings are the only animals who combine and mix various kind of food before eating and it is no coincidence that humans are only the animals who suffer from various digestive disorders.

How long to follow this Super Specialty Master Plan?

Within one month of following this Super Specialty Master Plan you will find most of the symptoms of your disease have already vanished, however in some chronic disease, it may take as much as 6 months of religious application of the Super Specialty Master Plan.

Since our aim is not just to recover from a specific illness, but to remain super fit and healthy lifelong, I recommend you to follow this plan lifelong. Make it a part of your lifestyle.

CHAPTER -NINETEEN

HOW TO MASTER ANY EMOTION

Emotions are feelings which can make you a king or a pauper in society. Whenever I feel painful emotions. I try to follow the following six steps and break my limiting patterns and not fall into the shackles of emotion. But I prefer to take a lesson from every emotion and purge myself from the pangs of emotions...

Let us understand these steps ...

STEP-1

People often feel overloaded by their emotions, without realizing their 'true' feelings. The sole thing they identify is some negativity, something wrong, something gloomy. I will suggest you to just put yourself into reverse gear and ask yourself" what exactly is troubling you? What are you feeling precisely? Try to pin down your emotions. Question yourself repetitively, "what am I feeling?" Irritated, hurt, harmed, rejected or something else. ...This exercise will lower your emotional passion you are feeling and will help to locate the problem. You will be able to deal with the situation more quickly, confidently and easily.

Say for example - Ask yourself "Am I feeling the pangs of separation" or "am I disappointed?" " or is somebody's success troubling me?"Or "Am I feeling cheated" "Is it just a phase or a serious problem?" Remember this questioning skill; this ability to transform an emotion in to a tangible expression, will immediately lower your intensity. Even more, it will make you to fight with a negative emotion with a triumph and learn from the experience.

How much has to be explored and discarded before reaching the naked flesh of feeling.

People don't try to show their feelings, they try to hide them.

The sign of intelligent people is their ability to control their emotions by the application of reasons.

Emotions are temporary state of mind, Don't let them destroy you permanently.

STEP-2

ACKNOWLEDGE AND VALUE YOUR EMOTIONS

Emotions are what drive us and also what drive us go astray. You cannot persuade yourself without understanding them well. Let's not forget that the little emotions are the great captains of our lives and we obey them without realizing it. We never want our emotions to be wrong. The moment we brand an emotion as 'wrong' kills the honest communication with ourselves. Emotions are our feelings. Literally, we feel them in our bodies as tingles, hot spots and muscular tension. These are cognitive aspects, but the physical sensation is what makes them really different. Never try to under rate your emotions, rather be thankful to them, as they are 'signaling' a change. A change in perception, action or processing a decision. Trust your emotions, even though you don't understand them, they will support you. Cherish your own emotions and never undervalue them. Labelling an emotion wrong will never lessen the intensity, as the maxim goes 'whatever you resist tends to persist'. Nurture a feeling of admiration for all emotions; they are like a crying child, who immediately calms down as soon as gets an attention.

STEP-3

FIGURE OUT THE MESSAGE - AN EMOTION IS OFFERING

Understand your emotions, try to find out what is it, whether it's tantrum or depression.

Emotions often lead to actions reflecting the emotion. When we feel something, we consequently respond to that feeling. This can be both in the immediate (and often subconscious) response to the feeling and also in the more thoughtful handling of the aftermath. Where this has been a negative feeling, the response may range from vigorous justification of our actions to conciliatory apologies and other 'making up'. A common response to the repression of unwanted emotions is displacement, where we act out our frustration in other ways. Thus a reprimanded child, knowing they cannot answer back, may go and 'punish' their toys.

Emotions affect and are also a part of our mood, which is usually a more sustained emotional state. Mood affects our judgment and changes how we process decisions.

So what? Get curious about your emotions, what are they really offering you . Ask yourself question, "What do I really want?"" What will I have to do to change my belief" "Am I misinterpreting the situatio" " Am I willing to create a solution and handle it right now?" "What do I learn from this"

So manage emotions. In negotiations, who gets his way is often the person who has the greatest emotional control.

STEP-4

GO AND GET IT

Be confident that you can deal with an emotion pretty well. I suppose it is the best, easy, nippiest and the most powerful way to handle any situation/ emotion. Try to recreate the magic of past, when a similar situation arose and you were able to handle it quite well, so YOU CAN DO IT again today. So, go in to the history and follow the dos and don'ts you performed. Use that as a role model to tackle the emotion. Say you felt rejected or thwarted or alienated, what did you then do to overcome it! Was it a visit to friend, a hug with someone close or hanging out with friends or was it an aerobic exercise. What did you do! Was your conception changed or your focus shifted...do the same, you will get the comparable results. Once you have understood those purging techniques or methods, these will always reproduce the analogous effects but always do it with a CONFIDENCE that YES IT WILL WORK…and no surprises! It will.

STEP- 5

ASSURE YOURSELF

Repeatedly tell yourself that I can handle this emotion today, tomorrow and whenever it comes. Rehearse the emotion again and again… feel, hear and react to the emotion…visualize yourself handling the situation 'easily'. This will create a neural pathway of belief that you can meet the challenges…a sort of conditioning…communicating yourself about the surety…try to enumerate the ways or steps that can change your perception when a red flag is seen. How you communicate your feelings …. how you change the actions and perceptions in a particular situation.

STEP-6

BE AN EXCITED COMBATANT AND STRIKE IT

Now when you have finished first five steps…i.e recognized the emotion, appreciated it, learnt what it was offering rather than dismissing it all together, comprehended how to bring ball to your court by modeling your reaction on past strategies and even rehearsed to combat a similar situation in future …… So the final step is ostensible ….. GET THRILLED AND TAKE ACTION. Express yourself as per the checklists you rehearsed to change the perception. Get excited to charter the vistas of emotions….

Just use these six steps and you can virtually master any… mind it… ANY emotional setback that comes up in your life. So, start practicing this system… Initially you may find it difficult or even cumbersome but soon you will be comfy with it. Like when you start with driving lessons..

changing gears, brakes ..accelerator all seem to be 'extraterrestrial' but with practice all happens effortlessly, involuntarily. Trust me your personal trainer will never let you down...It will guide you where to go and achieve your goal.. I would suggest to handle an emotion the moment you begin to feel it; it is easy to nip the evil in the bud rather than intervene it in a full blown state.

TEN BASIC EMOTIONS

With the six steps alone, you can change almost all emotions. But in order to keep yourself from even having to use these six steps, conscious understanding of positivity every emotion is offering will be useful to a great extent. I am going to share with you ten basic and primary emotions most people avoid but are having the potential to put you in action. Knowing these emotions won't give you instant mastery; you got to use these distinctions consistently to reap the remunerations. I would suggest you to read and reread this section and even pen down the action signals and carry along with you. This would be a constant reminder about the emotion, its true meaning for you and the suggested action plan for your utilization.

Let's begin with the most basic call to act...

1. DISCOMFORT

Uncomfortable emotions don't have the huge impact but constantly bother us and have a niggling sensation that 'all is not well'

Dismay, Disappointment, Displeasure Boredom, Despair, Hurt, Sadness, Boredom, Anxiety, tickles our nerve that all is not right. May be_____

But never mind the solution is simple

- Use the skills learnt previously
- Clarify your wants

- Refine and redefine your actions. Try a bit different strategy.

Like all feelings it has to be dealt with. Discomfort is painful but even more intense is the anticipation of pain or forthcoming danger. Here, I would like to say that our imagination can make a thing ten times more intense than the real situation. To quote Russell Green "Worry is a morbid anticipation of events which never happen". The feeling of being attacked is worse than the real attack. When we anticipate pain we start feeling another emotion and develop the signs of.......

2. FEAR

It is a distressing emotion induced by a perceived threat. Probably it is the oldest and strongest emotion of mankind. In words of Aristotle "Fear is pain arising from the anticipation of evil". *Anxiety, nervousness, tension, uneasiness, apprehension, worry, distress, dread they all signal that something is going to happen which needs an attention and preparation*. It is ironical that most of the people try to deny their fear or wallow in it. Neither of them is the right approach to deal with the emotion. You don't yield to fear and start thinking the worst or pretend its absence..in both the cases you are disrespecting the message, fear is trying to deliver.

Solutions for it, is easy. Firstly review your feelings and assess what must be done mentally. Enumerate the solutions or steps to deal with the situation . Sometimes it does happen that we've done what we could do but still fear persists. At this point you need to take an antidote, a pill for fear ...a 'faith pill'. You must decide to have faith in your preparation that this is all I could do. Mostly the fears which give us sleepless nights rarely come to fruition. Assure yourself that if at all they come ... you may experience.

3. HURT

It is the most widely felt emotion that rules the human relationships.

Almost all of us feel it personally, professionally and socially. It is generated by a sense of loss, a sense of being cheated, duped. The most common reaction is lashing out at others. But we need to listen to the message this feeling is giving us. We expect people to do something for us. Consciously and unconsciously, we feel hurt when somebody fails to meet our expectations. We expected somebody to keep a word or do something for us and if this doesn't happen we feel hurt, (even if we never told the concerned person about our expectations). This hurt feeling results in the experience of loss of love, intimacy and trust.

To overcome this feeling, just contemplate, you may not have lost anything, may be it is a false perception. May be what you perceive about the person is untrue, they may not be doing it purposely or realize the effect of their actions on you. Secondly, revaluate the situation. May be you are overreacting. Ask yourself "have I really suffered some loss" or "am I passing the judgment too soon".

The third step which will dilute your intensity (probably the most graceful and expressive way) is to communicate your feelings to the person concerned. Open your heart, be expressive and ask for an explanation.... Tell them "your abc statement / comment/action led me to think like this ..." You will happily discover that hurt disappears in moments. Remember, there is a thin line that separates laughter and pain, comedy and tragedy, humor and hurt.

4. ANGER

This hurt feeling, if not dealt transforms into anger. *Rage, outrage, fury, wrath, hostility, ferocity, bitterness, hate, scorn, spite, vengefulness, dislike, resentment* etc all are included in anger. This signals that, the yardsticks, standards fixed by you have been dishonoured and violated by you or someone else.

Try to understand that may be others are not aware of your parameters and set of laws (even though it was mandatory from your side) it means that you are misinterpreting the situation. Also you need to realize 'with a big heart' that may be the 'rules' set by you are not right.(what if you endorse them whole-heartily). Lastly ask yourself "Does the xyz person really cares about you and what should you do to make the person, know your standards", so that it is not repeated? So in nutshell, whenever you feel angry change your perception, review your rules and change your behavior and communicate to people what you expect of them.

If this emotion persists, it may lead to frustration ...

5. FRUSTRATION

This comes through many doors. Bottlenecks, Roadblocks, Barricades, *Depression, Despair, Hopelessness, Gloom, Glumness, Sadness, Unhappiness all precipitate to frustration. Continuous efforts in life seem to go futile, as if it has suddenly become a two side open pot and we tend to feel frustrated.*

But I may tell you if you are able to construe the message frustration is giving...you will be excited , rather enthralled... it says you could be doing much better than you are presently.

Imbibe the positive vibes this emotion is generating. It also reflects that solutions are within your range, you only need to change your approach, perception and turn out to be more adaptable and flexible.

To combat with it firstly be friends with frustration and devise new methods and ways to get results. Just try to flex your ideas and approach. Be creative and innovative, get some inputs from people who went through similar situation....a role model...tighten your belts to find a one for you. Accept the challenge, get fascinated by the situation and learn the lesson it is teaching you and equipping you for future .

6. DISAPPOINTMENT

It is demoralizing , disastrous and even devastating , if not dealt speedily .

The feeling of *despair, hopelessness, gloom, glumness......that you have or are going to miss something forever. In this one feel defeated, rejected, sad as the result is meagre as compared to expectations.*

But, there is also a ray of hope in it. It is offering you the opportunity to redefine your goal. The goal which you were running after will not materialize. So it is time to change your expectations and set a new goal instantly.

- *Immediately figure out what you can learn from this situation, that could help you in future.*

- *Set a new goal, even more attractive and inspiring and start with immediate effec.t*

- *Also, try to contemplate, that you are not judging the situation in haste........May be it is a passing phase. Remember God's delays are not God's denial.*

- *Lastly, all is not over, Re-evaluate the situation and develop a new effective plan......Develop a positive attitude for future.*

The ultimate disappointment we experience, it usually transforms into guilt.

7. GUILT

Emotions of guilt, regret, lament, remorse, penitence, repentance, shame are the feelings which we all do the most to avoid. These are indeed very painful to experience but definitely give a valuable message.

It says that you have violated some standards and you need to ensure that these are not repeated. Guilt is indeed painful but acts as leverage to change behaviour. Don't try to suppress it, as it never dies but comes back even stronger. But some may wallow in guilt and continue to experience the pain with a sense of catharsis and helplessness. This is not the message which guilt is giving us. It doesn't ask us to feel inferior, remorseful and lurch ourselves in continuous pain rather it signals to recommit yourself to higher standards once again.

For this.........

- Admit that you have violated a set standard.
- Commit to yourself that it will never happen again. Start a new with a recharged mind. Commit yourself beyond this.
- This is the purpose of guilt to drive you to higher standards.

But still there are some of us who manage to torture themselves mentally and emotionally, as they feel themselves to be incompetent to meet the standards and experiences.

8. INADEQUACY

When the feeling of insufficiency, dearth, unworthiness is experienced, we feel we should have had achieved something but can't do. We often have a completely unfair rule for determining whether we are inadequate or not ....but this is not all. We need to decipher the message it is offering.

It says that, presently you don't have necessary skill or competence, you need to have more information, strategies, tools and plans.

To overcome this feeling

- Just ask yourself , is this feeling of inadequacy true or is my perception wrong.
- Whenever this feeling strikes you, be motivated and appreciate the feeling of excellence and improvement.
- Find a role model, who is perfect in the area in which you feel inadequate. Get a, 'crash course' from him. You may be untrained or unskilled in that area but you are not inadequate. Don't lean yourself and get trapped in helplessness and self pity.

When some of us start feeling that problems are everlasting and pervasive and feel there are too many things to deal with in that case we succumb to.

9. OVERLOAD

Grief, misery, depression, helplessness are merely expressions of overload. When you feel like there is no empowering meaning for something happened and you feel your life is negatively impacted by people around and events. Things seem out of control and there is more going on than they can deal with ....

The message being flashed is that, you need to reevaluate, what is most important to you in the situation. May be you are dealing with lot of many things at a time with a feeling to change everything overnight. It can be really disruptive and destructive ....

To win over it:

- Decide what is most important for you .... focus on that.
- Pen down all the priorities, in descending order of priority .. You will see just writing them, only will give you a sense of control over them.
- Deal with the first in list and work on it till you have control over it, By doing this you will make your brain realize that you are not overloaded but have a control over things ....and the problem is not permanent.

We feel overloaded but forget that we also have the power to change this by focusing on what we can control and deal with it at a time.

10. LONELINESS

This feeling is feared the most.... A feeling of broken, disconnected, feeling alone and separated ... all belong to this.

Have you ever felt this .... I think almost all of us have experienced this some or the other time.....

The message it gives is that you need a connection with somebody. Often people misapprehend it as sexual intimacy .....but even after that they feel frustrated and still lonely ....

How to overcome it....

- Assure yourself that you can reach out and make a connection somewhere.... Believe it that there are caring people everywhere.

- Identify your need .... the connection you need .. may be you need a friend .. somebody to talk to ...to laugh..... a shoulder to cry...... so identify your need.

- Try to ponder over the undercurrent message it is offering that ' I love people..." I really care for them.....and want to be with them..." Trust me this is indeed a superior thing for a human .So reach out and find your needs.

- Connect with someone.... and cure the emotions. Here you are with the list of emotions...and Action signals, all offer you with empowering messages and call for a change which is sham and fake. It gives you a reason to dispel your negative perceptions, unsuitable procedures, your standards, your style and renew it. Look for the positive signals.

Nurture your garden of emotions, and your spirit as gardener... make it beautiful. Seed a bountiful of emotions like love, warmth, goodness, admiration than the crop of negative feelings of anger and fear, disappointment. Reap a harvest of healthier plants ....keep cultivating the plants (emotions) you need and keep pulling the weeds timely. Your life will flourish and fulfil the highest potential......Hold youself to a standard of greatness ....

CHAPTER -TWENTY

HOW TO MAINTAIN A LONG TERM SUPER HEALTH?

Technique to maintain long term super health:

As we know that going to a gym just once or twice will not ensure a lifetime fitness, similarly following the Super Specialty Master Plan just once or twice will not ensure a disease free life. We have to make it a part of our life. We have to commit it to our habit. The main question is "How to make it a habit" Remember, *repetition is the mother of a habit*. Doing just once or twice will not serve the purpose. We must repeat the process number of times, so as to make it a part of the habit. For that we have to remind ourselves several times in a day, about the benefits of following the same and also the demerits of not following it.

I can help you to create a mental reminder system, which will constantly remind you about the intrinsic worth of this diet plan. I call the system as memory watch. We have to create a memory watch in the mind or in the physical form.

Step 1: Read the dial of the Memory Watch.

Step 2: Memorize the dial. You will be able to do it in just 3 to 5 minutes as the word associated with each of the numbers, rhyme with the number.

In this method numbers are represented by a thing or an image and we have to ensure that the name of these things rhyme with the number.

The usual rhyming scheme is given as follows:

One rhymes with Sun

Two rhymes with Shoe

Three rhymes with Tree

Four rhymes with Door

Five rhymes with Knife

Six rhymes with Kicks

Seven rhymes with Heaven

Eight rhymes with Plate

Nine rhymes with Wine

Ten rhymes with Hen

Eleven rhymes with Lemon

Twelve rhymes with Shelve

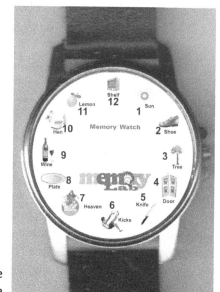

Now say we have to remember the following appointments for the day:-

1'O Clock	:	Go to the airport to receive a friend
3'O Clock	:	Go to the birthday party
4'O Clock	:	Music classes
6'O Clock	:	Shopping
7'O Clock	:	Internet café
8'O Clock	:	Go for the dance class
9'O Clock	:	Taking the car for servicing
10'O Clock	:	Going for the tuition
12'O Clock	:	Meeting with the Chief Minister

To remember the above appointment list you simply have to associate it with the picture of corresponding time. For e.g.

3 O' Clock (Tree): Go for the birthday party

(Tree) Imagine that you are celebrating the birthday on the tree.

7 O' Clock(Heaven): Internet Café

(Heaven) Imagine gods and goddesses are surfing the net in the heaven.

8 'O' Clock (Plate): Dance Classes

(Plate) Imagine yourself dancing on a big sized plate.

4 O' Clock (Door): Music Classes

(Door) Imagine instead of a tabla, you are using door to play music.

9 O' Clock (Wine): Servicing of the car

(Wine) Imagine in the filling station, your car is being refueled with wine instead of petrol.

10 O' clock (Hen) : Tuition

(Hen) Imagine a hen is taking tuition classes for you.

12 O' Clock (Shelve) : Meeting with the Chief Minister

(Shelve) Imagine the Chief Minister is sitting on a shelf during the meeting.

Or if you want to recall at what time!

You have to go for the dance classes. The very thought of dance will help you recall plate which will indicate the time as 8 O'clock.

Now next time you need to recall what you need to do at 3 O' clock just by focusing on the rhyming word of 3 i.e. tree and you will be able to recall the birthday party. In case you need to recall at what time you need to go for shopping. The visual of shopping will help you recall the time for that.

This is usually a temporary memory and once the task or appointment is over this memory will automatically fade away.

Once you learn all the 12 rhyming codes, this method will become very handy to remember small day to day activities such as appointments, shopping lists or even important points of a speech, in case you have to deliver one.

Now you are prepared with the memory watch. The memory watch is there in your mind. For greater impact you can make your own memory watch by replacing the connotational dial of your watch with those 12 rhyming words or you can contact us.

How to use the memory watch to remind ourselves of the important things to do for a perfect health!

Important points to remember and comply for a perfect health:

1. Lots of raw vegetables in diet.

2. 8 to 10 glasses of water from copper jug.

3. Watching laughter videos to create a positive harmony among the organs for quick healing.

4. Maintain alkaline pH balance.

5. Banishing white poison (refined sugar, milk, refined flour, processed rice and table salt).

6. No to packed/processed food.

7. Exercise, Exercise, Exercise at least one hour per day.

8. Positive attitude for positive result.

9. Guided mental imagery for quick relief from illness.

10. Maintaining a regular routine of 6 to 8 hrs of sleep as body does most of maintenance and building work during the sleep time.

11. Wheatgrass Therapy.

12. Lots of fresh fruit diet.

Step 3: Now you are prepared to memorize small sequence of appointments with the help of the Memory Watch.

Let's say you want to remember the following appointment for the day (Refer Page-141 Super Specialty Time Table)

- At 1:00 O'clock, visualize that Sun is eating raw vegetables in a big platter.

- At 3:00 O'clock, visualize that on a tree laughing videos are running on a TV and you are laughing after watching it.

- At 7.00 O'clock, visualize that in heaven all gods are exercising.

- At 10 .00 O'clock, visualize that a hen is sleeping and snoring loudly.

- At 12.00 O'clock, visualize that you are decorating lots of colorful fruits on the shelf.

CHAPTER -TWENTY ONE

SUPER SPECIALTY- WEIGHT LOSS AND SIX PACK ABS

W hy some people are fat?

People generally associate excess fat with excess quantity of food intake. But the truth is it's not the quantity of food that matters it the QUALITY OF INTAKE which matters the most. When I say intake....

It means 1. What do we think.
2. What do we eat.

Let's Focus On Four Top Reasons Of Fat Accumulation

1. Stress:

If a person is living for years in a state of unresolved anger towards a spouse or child or family member, or a person works for the years under a pressure of boss or a system that makes him/her powerless and abused, that person may experience a constant anger or a sense of danger.

This long term stress, in fact any stress long or short, causes a steady flow of stress hormone called Cortisol (higher and more prolonged levels of Cortisol in the bloodstream have negative effects, like: Suppressed Thyroid Function.

Blood Sugar imbalances (such as Hyperglycemia, Decreased Bone Density, Higher Blood Pressure, Lowered Immunity and Inflammatory responses in the body, Slow Wound Healing, many more health consequences) the blood stream and it can be very damaging for the body. Too much of

Cortisol can make the body gain weight especially in the mid section of the body.

2. Excessive Acidic Food:

Calories in the food items are not the only reason for weight gain and obesity will not work in general in this case. Healthy weight is directly related to the alkalinity and acidity in our food.

$$\text{Excess Calories} \neq \text{Excess Weight}$$

$$\text{Excess Acidic Food} = \text{Excess Weight}$$

Your body works valiantly to keep the excess of acid or acidic environment, away from your vital organs (Losing this battle is why there are so many heart attacks and strokes). What your body must do is find a place to stick that acid, and so it goes into your fat cells, as fat is a pretty good medium to keep acid away from the organs.

When fat cells fill, a person gets fatter, and looks bloated. Even thin people with acidic imbalance often get "puffy" looking.

The effectiveness with which your nervous system can operate is subject to a correct pH.

3. Excessive Salt Intake:

Excessive Salt in the body also increases the weight of the body because of the following reasons. Kidneys eliminate excess salt from the body by filtering out the sodium that makes up part of the salt. In case kidneys work less efficiently either because they have gone weak or because of lowered blood supply to them (because of weak heart), the kidneys excrete sodium less efficiently and more sodium is retained in the body. Since the kidneys are geared to maintain a fixed proportion of sodium to water in the blood, excess salt in the body means excess water too and it leads to excess weight of the body.

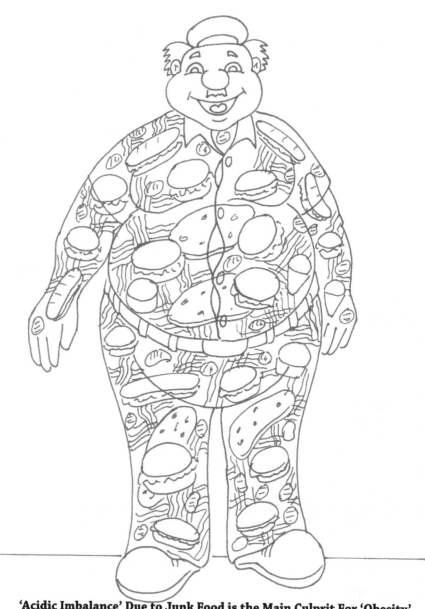

'Acidic Imbalance' Due to Junk Food is the Main Culprit For 'Obesity'

4. Dead Food:

If you want to lose fat and calcium deposited in your joints, cholesterol in your arteries or break down cancerous tumor. It is the enzymes, from the living food, which will perform these functions. Dead or processed food like pizza, burger, pastries, chips all are devoid of enzymes.

By eliminating the above 4 causes (Stress, Excess acidic food, Excess salt intake and dead food) of getting excess fat in the body, we will not only be able to lose weight, but also weigh in right proportion, our body will look symmetrical......just like film stars.

Before we get into the "details" of the training techniques and dietary strategies for losing belly fat and getting those six pack abs, I want to show you the #1 reason why most people fail to achieve this goal.

If you ignore this starting point, it is most likely that you will never get the fitness results that you're looking for. This explains why so many people struggle back and forth with their fitness for years and years of frustration.

The #1 reason for failure to achieve their fitness goal in the most people, is the general procrastination, laziness, and poor mental attitude about what they BELIEVE they can actually achieve.

The #2 reason for failure fat loss & achieving their dream body is ineffective training routines and poor dietary habits.

The reason I put, mental attitude and beliefs before the actual details of training/nutrition for weight loss is because your mental status is the true starting point for success in anything.

This involves:

1. DECIDING exactly what do you want (how do you want your body to look, how much confidence do you want to feel, how much energy do you want, internal health, etc.)

2. Make sure you actually have a BURNING DESIRE for what you want to achieve.

3. Setting/documenting EXACT GOALS for what you want to achieve.

4. VISUALIZING and "FEELING" what you want to achieve, as if you have already achieved it.

5. BELIEVING that you CAN actually achieve it.

6. Taking massive action NOW to start achieving (no procrastination).

In order to ever be successful at anything, all excuses need to go out of the window... there is no such thing as poor genetics, no such thing as "not enough time", no such thing as "it's just too hard"... no excuses at all for not achieving what you set out to achieve.

This is the stuff nobody ever wants to talk about, but this is more important and should be set right before dealing with the "details" about workouts and how to eat for fat loss or any goal for that matter.

So make sure to take a 2nd look at those 6 aspects (given above) of your mindset, that you should absolutely be clear about first. I want you to really give some serious thought to each one of them above.

Once you're straight on the type of mindset that it's going to take to achieve this goal, then you can get started to the next step.

Healthiest Way to Weight Loss:

To eliminate the above 4 reasons (stress, excess acidic food, excess salt intake and dead food) and to reduce weight in a healthiest way is to follow the Super Specialty Master Plan for few months. Since our aim is not to be zero sized or super thin, which is very dangerous for the body, as it invites lots of serious diseases. We would like to remain in the perfect shape with lots of energy and vitality long life. Once you see the effectiveness of Super Specialty Master Plan after few months of religious implemention I am hopeful...in fact I can bet...that you would like to follow Super Specialty Master Plan long life.

How to Have Six Pack Abs:

We all are born with six pack abs, but for the most of us ....we need a detective to find it ....that is hidden under the belly. On an average one in one lakh people, is having a visible six pack abs.

They are not limited to only Shahrukh, Amirs Khan and Hritik Roshans ...all can get them...you too can have them only you need to follow

Two steps to have a visible six pack.

Step I: Reduce the excess fat deposits. For that the best way is to follow SSMP for 6 months to start with.

Step II: Physical excersice targeting the specific area of the body, will lead to a six pack abs.

I am suggesting you here a set of 6 powerful exercises. Doing it for few months along with the SSMP will lead to a six pack abs.

EXERCISE 1:
Lying Leg Thrusts

This is a two part exercise – a "halfway down" leg raise followed by a hip thrust. Start by lying on your back with your head and shoulders raised off of the floor, your hands (palms down) on the mat by your hips, and your legs at a 90° angle from the floor. Slowly lower your legs only half way to the floor to an angle of approximately 45° from the floor. Do not go all the way to the floor with the legs as this promotes an arched back and can put a lot of stress on the lumbar spine. From the 45° position, raise your legs back

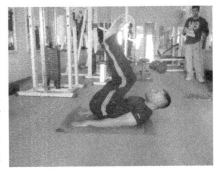

up to the 90° position. Once the legs are back at the 90° position (no further), thrust your hips off the floor.

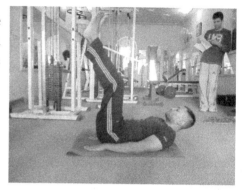

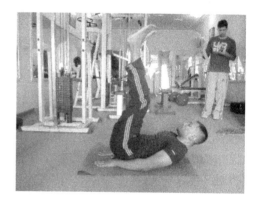

EXERCISE 2:

Reverse Crunches

Start by lying on your back on a mat with your feet flat on the floor, your knees at a 90° angle, and your palms on the floor by your hips, and your head and shoulders slightly lifted off the ground. Slowly crunch your lower body off the ground by

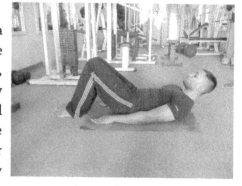

curling your pelvis back toward your head. Do not use momentum. Rather, use your abdominal strength to perform the movement.

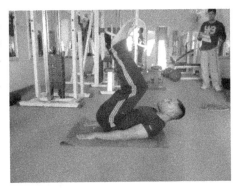

EXERCISE 3:

Abdominal Bicycles

Start by lying on your back on a mat with both your hips and your knees at 90° angles and your head and shoulders slightly lifted off the ground with your fingers touching the sides of your head (not pulling on the back of your head). Perform the movement by crunching the left side of your upper body off the floor and bringing your left elbow and right knee together simultaneously. Then extend your right knee out and bring your right elbow and left knee together simultaneously. This

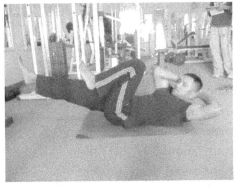

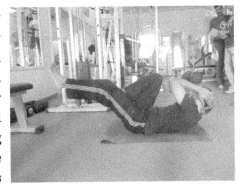

ends up almost mimicking a bicycling movement in a lying position, except keeping your legs moving in and out linearly instead of cyclically.

EXERCISE 4:

Abdominal Scissors

Start by lying on your back on a mat with both your arms straight back over your head and your legs straight out at about a 45° angle from vertical. Bring your shoulders off the ground and arms forward while simultaneously bringing your legs and hips up off the ground such that your legs and arms slightly cross over.

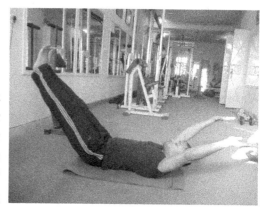

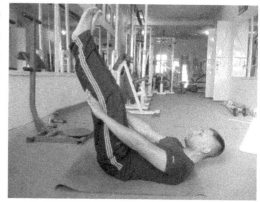

EXERCISE 5:

Bench Crunches

This is still the basic upper body crunching movement; however, your lower legs will be up on a bench with both the knees and hips at 90°angles and your back flat on the mat. With your fingers on the sides of your head, crunch your upper body up bringing your elbows towards your knees. To get the best results, focus on holding the top position of the crunch for two seconds while forcefully exhaling and holding a hard contraction of the abs.

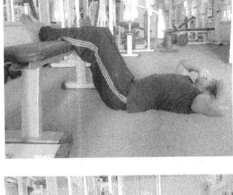

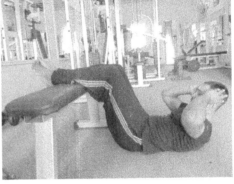

Spend about ½ an hr doing a combination of the above exercises, six days a week. Try to increase the speed of exercise along with time also.

CHAPTER -TWENTY TWO

WHEATGRASS AND BODYBUILDING

In the previous chapter you read about different ways of weight loss and techniques to develop six pack abs. Let's now read about contribution of Wheatgrass in bodybuilding.

1. Wheatgrass is a herbal element rich in amino acids. The body uses amino acids to build protein and protein to build muscles. Wheatgrass, as a dietary supplement, also provides vitamins, minerals and chlorophyll, which work to improve the immune system.

2. Building strength requires a full routine that exercises the key muscle groups. Wheatgrass is a natural supplement that contains essential elements for growth and enhances your strength training.

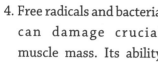

3. Physical training increases oxidative stressing in the body, and this increased stress may lead to immune system suppression and over-training. Wheat grass can help speed recovery and support health because of its antioxidant effect.

4. Free radicals and bacteria can damage crucial muscle mass. Its ability

to stimulate red blood cell production aids in the building of muscle tissue, and wheatgrass is thus ideal for the hard training athlete. Anabolic steroids act to increase protein synthesis via an increase in red blood cell production, and is responsible for increase in muscle tissue.

5. Wheatgrass' ability to protect the immune system makes it an ideal supplement pre and post workout. Muscle tissue is most vulnerable to exercise-induced oxidative damage post-workout, and muscular repair cannot occur in the presence of free radicals. As a free antioxidant wheatgrass will scavenge your system for free-radicals, ensuring that you grow as much as possible from your workout.

Ingest one dose of wheatgrass after a workout. This supplement will help your body heal and utilize the workout to build muscle Take small dosages of wheatgrass juice throughout the day, target dose 80 to 100 ml of wheatgrass a day will help overall health and supplement a balanced diet. Take the wheatgrass on an empty stomach for best result.

Christian Bale transformed his body from a severely underweight 54 kg to a bulky 99.79 kg in around 5 months to play as superfit super hero in the Hollywood movie *Batman Begins*. Intensive bodyweight workouts, resistance/weight training workouts and diet played an important role in such an intensive training regime. Meals having a good balance of quality protein sources, and carbs in the form of salads, vegetables fruits and wheatgrass juice played an important role in achieving this.

CHAPTER -TWENTY THREE

SUPER SPECIALTY FIRST AIDS AND BEAUTY TIPS

Beauty lies in the eyes of the beholder. Remember nothing in particular is beautiful or ugly in this world. It is only the perception of it. For every mother, the most beautiful face on earth is the face of her child.

The first principle to be beautiful to the world is to feel and believe that you are beautiful. Let's understand the science behind it. Stand in front of a mirror. Try to pick up one aspect of your look, which you like the most and want it to be comparatively more beautiful in future.

Feel good about it. Similarly try to pick some more physical or behavioral aspects of yourself, which you love very much and offer your gratitude to the God for gifting you all those good features and qualities. Now let's understand what happens in the brain:

Step 1: We decide to feel good about ourselves .

Step 2: Enjoy the feel- good moment.

Step 3: Brain registers the feeling.

Step 4: Brain stimulates the production of happy hormone.

Step 5: Happy hormone triggers a sequence of activities like energising the body, sparkling in the eyes, erect posture, and more active outlook, shining hair, odorless mouth, healthy skin texture and a smile on the face.

Step 6: Resulting in the more beautiful you.

Now you know that even the best cosmetic in the world will not work for you, unless you really feel good about yourself from inside.

The truth about cosmetics: The most beautiful thing in this world is watching a smiling baby. The beauty in the child's face is not because of the application of expensive cosmetics.

Some Facts about Man-Made Cosmetics

1. No cosmetic has been invented which can make you fairer.

2. No cosmetic can eliminate wrinkles permanently from your face.

3. No cosmetic can cure the pimple or acne.

The cosmetic can mask the symptoms or can give a temporary make-up, but it cannot enhance the beauty.

Repeated usage of cosmetic for a definite period of time can lead to the permanent damage to the skin (remember the skin of face is more delicate than the skin of any other part of the body).

Abandon all kinds of cosmetics which you might be using and go for the following solutions for your every need related to skin and first aid.

BEAUTY TIPS

1. FACE MASK

You will need:

2 tablespoons honey

2 teaspoons milk

Method:
Mix the honey with milk. Smooth over the face and throat. Leave for 10 minutes before rinsing off with warm water.

2. SKIN SOFTENING BATH

For a classically simple treat, try adding three or four tablespoons of honey to the bath water. You will enjoy silky fragrant bath.

3. HAIR CONDITIONER

You will need:

120ml honey

2 tablespoons olive oil

Mix honey and olive oil. Give a smooth coating to the hair with this mixture. Cover the hair and Leave or 30 minutes. Shampoo well and rinse.

4. SKIN EXFOLIATE

You will need:

1 tablespoon ground Oats
1 full tablespoon ground Almonds
1 tablespoon Honey
1 tablespoon fresh Aloe Vera gel

Method:

First of all, keep all the ingredients in a big bowl and gently mix them. Apply this mixture on the face and neck before performing toning and after cleansing. The person should apply this mixture by using his hands in circular motions. When the mixture gets dried, then one should rinse it off with lukewarm water. This mixture should be applied only after using facial mask.

To improve a Dull and Greasy Complexion:

- Mix half teaspoon of lime juice with one teaspoon of cucumber juice and a few drops of rose water. Apply it on the face and neck and leave it for 15 minutes. Wash off with lukewarm water.

5. SKIN TONER:

You will need:

3 to 4 cotton balls
2 tablespoon Aloe Vera gel

First of all, a cotton ball should be soaked in an aloe vera gel and then apply it on the face to eliminate excess oil and provides freshness to the skin. One can apply this after moisturizer and can use it daily. It is perfect for normal and oily skin. If one is having sensitive skin, then the gel should be divided into 50 – 50 ratio along with spring water. Aloe Vera juice can also be applied directly in case of sensitive skin.

6. SMOOTHING SKIN LOTION

1 teaspoon Honey
1 teaspoon vegetable oil
1 teaspoon Lemon juice

Method:

Mix all the ingredients together. Rub into hands, elbows, heels and any other areas of dry skin. Leave for 10 minutes. Rinse off with warm water.

7. LONGEVITY, STAYING YOUNG AND PREVENT GRAYING AND FALLING OF HAIR

You will need:

2-3 Amla per day

Method: Extract the juice of Amla (50ml), drink it for 31 days every year.

8. FOR RADIANT AND GLOWING SKIN:

Continuous consumption of Tulsi leaves extract with honey taken for 48 days, will improve the complexion and bring radiance and glow.

9. FOR TIGHTENING THE SKIN:

Semi dried Wheatgrass (left after the extraction of juice) can be dipped in the Wheatgrass juice and can be applied to the skin for tightening the loose and saggy skin.

10. FOR PIMPLES:

Gently apply a lemon peel on the pimples, leave for 15 minutes before washing it off.

- Pimples can be cured within a week, if radish leaves juice is applied on it.

11. THE GREATEST COSMETIC:

The beauty of wearing a smile cannot be compared with any cosmetics of the world. Research proves that smile and laughter produces ₹ 10,000/- worth of endorphin in the body leading to an enhancement in the mood, positivity of the mind and makes the person charming and loveable to the people around him/her.

FIRST AID SECTION

- **For Hiccups:** Take a piece of fresh lemon and suck it to cure the hiccups.

- **For Mouth Sores (Cankers):** In a glass of lukewarm water, mix the juice of a freshly squeezed lemon. Rinse your mouth frequently with this solution at least thrice a day.

- **For Belching:** Consume undiluted juice of one medium sized lemon twice a day. You can take it every day till you find relief.

- **For Eczema:** Take basil leaves to get 2-3 tablespoons of it, add juice of 1 lemon and a teaspoon of honey, apply this on affected areas.

- **For Hangover:** Mix together the juice of 4 lemons, 3 tablespoons vinegar, in 2 cups of lukewarm water and drink it.

- **For Insect Bites:** Add 20 drops of lemon oil to a cup of water and use it as an insect-repellent spray.

- **For Sprain:** Incorporating pineapple in your diet has shown the ability to get relief from sprains.

- **For Sunburn:** Apply cucumber juice to the affected parts for relief.

- **For Itching from Ring-Worm:** Holy basil leaves can be eaten for removal of worms.

- **For Prickly Heat:** You can apply the gram flour paste on the affected area.

- **For Nose bleeding:** Squeeze out some fresh lemon juice. Soak a cotton bud in it and gently dab inside of your nose, tilting your head slightly forward to prevent the blood from flowing into the throat. Injured blood vessels contract as soon as they come into contact with lemon juice.

- **For Bites and Stings:** Apply crushed garlic to the bites and stings areas.

- **For Animal Bites:** Mix some crushed garlic cloves in warm water, wash the wound with it thoroughly and then keep a moist compress on it.

- **For Food Poisoning:** Take three cloves of garlic and an equivalent amount of ginger simmered ten minutes in water and should be divided into two doses. Consume it in morning and evening.

- **For High Blood Pressure:** Consume 1 to 3 garlic cloves.

- **For Palm Burning Sensation:** Grind a handful of bitter gourd leaves into a smooth paste and apply on the affected areas of feet and palms frequently.

- **For Stomach Heaviness:** Mix 1 tsp powdered cumin and black pepper in a glass of buttermilk. Drink 2 to 3 times a day for 2-3 days.

- **For Thorn Removal:** If the thorn is not coming out then simply mix jaggery(gur) and carom seeds (ajwain) and tie on it. The thorn will come out itself only.

- **For Vomiting Due to Indigestion:** Take lemon juice frequently.

- **Stomach ache:** Stomach ache caused after meals and gas trouble is cured by drinking the mixture of lemon juice and radish juice.

- **For Broken Bone:** By eating garlic buds, after frying it in ghee relieves the fracture pain.

- **For Loose Stools:** Loose stools can be stopped by drinking carrot juice.

- **For Dog Bites:** If a dog bites then by applying garlic paste on it. Moreover boiling garlic paste in water and drinking it and having more garlic in meal (at least for seven days) destroys the poisonous effect.

- **For Weakness:** By drinking carrot juice, body gets instant strength and weakness vanishes.

A glass of beetroot juice as well as carrot juice can also reduce general weakness and refresh you.

- **Fever and Flu:** Fever and flu can be cured by drinking onion juice repeatedly.

  Daily occurring fever is avoided by drinking decoction of mint and ginger juice.

- **For Motion Sickness:** In case of giddiness, keep cinnamon clove in the mouth.

- **For Headache:** Headache can be cured after drinking coconut water.

- **For Sunburns:** Aloe Vera is quite effective in sunburns. Apply directly aloe vera gel on the effective parts.

- **For Hiccups:** (already in book on pg 174) but this one is juice therapy Hiccups can be stopped by drinking radish juice.

- **To Relieve Tired Eyes:** Take four tablespoons each of lime juice and iced water. Saturate cotton pads in this water and place over your closed eyelids for 10 minutes.

- **For Mouth Ulcers:** Prepare Aloe Vera mouthwash by mixing Aloe Vera juice and water. Use this mouthwash three times a day to speed up the healing of mouth ulcers.

- **For Relaxing Foot:** Lemon can be used for foot relaxation. You can soak your feet in warm water and rub them with lemon juice. This action will open the pores and moreover lemon juice provides a cooling effect. This treatment is said to promote better sleep, because of its relaxing action on the foot nerves.

First Aid through Wheat Grass Juice Only

For Eyes:
Wheatgrass juice has wonderful applications for the eyes problems. Use only one or two drops in the eye, for eye strain and tension. Because of its

richness in magnesium, wheatgrass acts as a smooth muscle relaxant.

For Ears:

Apply the Wheatgrass juice with a dropper in affected ear. It helps to reduce the pressure and discomfort of any type of ear ache.

For Nose:

Put one or two filtered drops with a dropper of Wheatgrass juice. It reduces inflamed nasal passages and soothes mucous membranes irritated from allergies.

For Cold or Sore Throat:

Gargle with the filtered wheat grass juice at the first sign of a cold or sore throat.

For Bad Breath:

Wheatgrass juice is also a great mouthwash and leaves your breath smelling fresh even after eating garlic. Bleeding gums, trench mouth, pyorrhea, bleeding and gingivitis, any gum problems in general are very responsive to Wheatgrass. For that you can chew the Wheatgrass or rub on the affected area.

For Sleeping Disorder:

Place a tray of living wheat grass near the head of your bed. It will enhance the oxygen in the air and generate healthy negative ions to help you sleep more soundly. Other way is to take Wheatgrass juice before bedtime.

For Asthma and Bronchitis:

Put semi dried wheat grass (left after the extraction of juice) on the back and chest. You can also drink Wheatgrass juice because it gives you relief.

CHAPTER -TWENTY FOUR

TESTIMONIALS

A New Beginning:

Now the truth is in front of you and it's time to convert it into action. Most of the people after getting all this knowledge say "it's a great eye opener but...... it does not fit into my lifestyle". Remember one thing dear, you can have lifestyle only when you will have life.

Q. How to take the first step?

Answer: Everything starts with a thought. Nothing happens, unless first you have thought about it, in the mind. For example you don't love to eat anything without thinking about it. You really have to think of the past pleasurable memory of eating a burger or a pizza or an ice-cream. You have to recall the taste, the smell and the picture of it. As a result you recreate the desire to have it again.

Steps of Redesigning Food Habit

Step 1: Decide what is ultimately a nourishing food for you.

Step 2: Create a mental picture of all the benefits of eating it, including how you will look 6 months from now after following the changed diet plan,... Your energy level, getting rid of all kinds of physical pains which you might be facing, because of your present garbage (junk) food habits etc.

Step 3: Mentally try to see it vividly with colours and in very big size. Try to take some time, while visualizing this.

Step 4: Feel the desire of the food and immediately convert your healthy desire into action.

A Rebellious Child: Know that you are the master of your thoughts. No one else, but only you can control what goes inside your head. As we are trying to change our diets or lives in general, we often experience resistance to that change.

For Example: If you had a little child, who was allowed to stay up, as late as he/she wanted for a long time. Then one day you make a decision that now you want your child to go to bed at 8:00 p.m. every night, what do you think the first night would be like!

Many times the child will rebel against this new rule kicking, screaming, fighting, or whatever else he/she may do to stay up late. If you give in at this time, the child wins and will try to control you forever.

However, if you firmly, yet calmly stick to your decision that this is the new bedtime, the rebellion will lessen. In two to three nights you will establish a new routine.

The mind works the same way. Often our brain is adapted to certain eating/thinking habits. It doesn't want to be retrained. Sometimes as we make new decisions or rules for our life, that little child pops up in our brain showing great resistance. But you are the master of your thoughts, thoughts are in your control. If you will stay focused and firm about your decisions, you will establish in a very short time, a new way of thinking, over time, gradually set some rules, stick to them, and re-train your inner child.

Take Responsibility: Remember whatever/whoever you are, is the result of your past action. Your today's physical or mental health is the result of a series of actions and habits of the past. It never happened in a moment. It takes 15 years of persistent smoking for a chain smoker to develop cancer, so it should take some time and effort to reverse it.

It's like going to a gym. You don't go to gym just once and say now I am fit for life time. After little time and dedication your muscles grow and adapt to a new change. So take time and be good to yourself. If you are suffering from some chronic ailment, then it should take about 3-6 months to see a significant difference in your physical/mental health and eventually you would come to love the 'Super Specialty Master Plan' and never want to return to a junk food life style.

And finally have some patience, as we know when we have junk food, there is no immediate symptoms of a disease although the damaging process by the junk food, starts in the body from the very first bite. It takes some amount of damage before the symptoms appear. Similarly the S^2MP will start working from the very moment you start implementing it but it will take some time to see a remarkable recovery from the disease.

I end this with a hope that it will bring a new beginning in you.

Testimonial: It has been seen that in many cases, the patient gets disheartened as they could not cure themselves with the conventional medicine and after years of suffering and in some cases after being shown doors by the modern hospitals, patients take this nature's route as the last resort. I suggest it to be the only option. I can say this with conviction as I am one of the beneficiary of the Natural Healing System.

My Story: I was born with a hole in my heart and as a result was always sick. At the age of 4 yrs the hole was diagnosed and doctors suggested for an open heart surgery although the survival chances in that was only 50%. The operation was successfully done to fill the hole of heart but doctors advised that for the entire life, I should avoid giving much strain to my body and to stay away from any kind of strenuous, physical activities including physical sports etc. As a result till the college days, I was only a silent observer during all sports activities around.

In year 1998, I came across a book on Mind Healing and came to know the power of mind. Using the power of mind not only I could heal myself completely but also broke world record of Canadian body builder who had completed 138 push-ups in one minute. I broke his record by doing 198 push-ups in one minute.

The Story that Inspires me the Most: October 2, 1996 Lance Armstrong was diagnosed with lungs and testicular cancer and brain tumour. Doctors predicted that his chances of survival are less than 40% and even if he survives he will never be able to lead a normal life. He proved it wrong by curing himself of the diseases and winning Tour-De-France (most grueling cycling championship) Championship for seven times. In his journey to success wheat grass juice and mind power played an important role.

Now this power within is with you and right now you are holding in your hand the training manual, which can guide you towards a superior you.

Some Success Stories of the People who Used the Powers of Nature:

<u>CANCER (colon)</u>
Snigdha Rane, (Female patient, Age 47 Yrs.), Lucknow

I was under radiotherapy after being operated for colon cancer. I faced lot of side effects such as hair loss, weakness, burning sensation, swelling of the body, etc. I had almost lost all the hope. Then I came to know about Dr. Biswaroop Roy Chowdhury's DISEASE REVERSAL seminar to be held in Lucknow...despite my poor health I decided to attend his seminar...there I learnt how wheatgrass can help me cure my cancer and regain my health back...I started taking wheatgrass juice twice a day...

Within 3 months it benefited me by easing away my side effect problems due to radiotherapy and my reports also showed me regaining normal health. I felt energetic and could lead a normal lifestyle...

WEIGHT LOSS
Sudeep Gupta (Male patient, age 45 Yrs Weight 116 Kg.), Pune

I was facing lot of health problems due to being over-weight. After taking lot of various treatments to reduce weight, I finally decided to try Wheatgrass therapy.

In order to reduce weight, diet has to be reduced. Many at times, the drastic reduction in nutritional foods causes other health hazards too. This increases the craving for foods and the weight reduction plan fails. I attended Dr. Biswaroop's Behaviour Modification Seminars. There I learnt how my bad habits can be modified into healhy habits and how food cravings can be dealt with effectively using Neuro Linguistic Programming...I then started on wheatgrass juice as advised by Dr Roy in the morning, empty stomach... Wheatgrass supplements the body's nutrition requirement even if the diet is reduced. It gives a feeling of fullness and reduces hunger pangs. The balanced nutrients promote the body to lose excess fats and reduce weight. Wheatgrass therapy and mild exercise, Within 3 months I reduced 10 Kg and further reduced 16 kg in next 7 months. I could reduce a total of 26 kgs in 10 to 12 months. .

SKIN PROBLEM

Chetna Anand (Female patient, Age 29 Yrs.), Pimpri

I had severe itching and irritation on many body parts. Even my face had turned ugly due to the continuous scratching of the skin. I tried lots of medication but got temporary relief. I got cured in three months when I started drinking wheatgrass juice on a regular basis.

THALASSEMIA

Simmi Kapur M/O Kunal kapur(Male child, Age 6 Yrs.), Moga

My child started having fits and recurring fever. Various treatments did not result into improvements. Testing of blood samples revealed that the production of blood in his body was inadequate. There was no solution to this problem other than giving blood transfusion at required intervals.

My child was given transfusion every fifteen days. Fed up of the agony our child was undergoing, we approached Dr. Biswaroop to know about Wheatgrass as an alternative therapy and immediately started the course,He also provided us wheatgrass juicer to make our work easy.... Within six months his blood transfusion could be skipped as the blood production improved. After another few months, the requirement for blood transfusion was reduced to negligible. After this Kunal was kept on maintenance dose for 3 months after which his condition was noted almost normal...now he requires just 4 to 5 transusions in a year with the number of transfusions decreasing every year....

PILES and ARTHRITIS

Govind kumar Verma (Male patient, Age 86 Yrs.), Ghaziabad

I had severe piles problem for last few years. I also suffered from insomnia, loss of appetite, gases, arthritis, etc. Medicines were giving only mild relief. I started looking for alternate therapy to relieve me from this endless suffering. Then I along with my 47 yr old son attended Dr Roy's Health Seminar in Dehradun and came to know about miracles of wheatgrass. Me and my son started drinking Wheatgrass morning and evening. All my health problems were reduced within two months of the Wheatgrass therapy and, my son remains energetic throughout the whole day and is as healthy as any 30 yr old.. Most importantly, my piles were completely cured. Now I feel better and even at this age I can independently take care of my daily chores.

DIABETES

Raghubir Singh(male PATIENT, AGE 69 Yrs.), Kaithal

I was a prosperous business 3 of 123 and the Hemoglobin count also increased to 12, which is normal level. Now I feel energetic and can go for walks. It's been more than a year now I am maintaining good health...and I am more prosperous...because I got both, health and wealth.....

ARTHRITIS
Indira Desai (Female patient, Age 78 Yrs.), Shimla

I used to have severe knee pain and had skin pigmentation on the face due to old age. I was taking medicines over a considerable duration but the problems were persistent. Then I started taking Wheatgrass juice along with the treatment and it helped me to solve both the problems within 3 months from starting it. Now I can walk freely without any knee pain and the skin on my face is cleared of the pigmentation...

LOW HEART BEAT
Sunita Bali (Female patient, Age 27 Yrs.), Sriharikota

A normal healthy person's heart beat count is 72 to 80 per minute. My heartbeats were around 50 per minute. This caused anemia, weakness, giddiness, and my weight dropped to 41 Kg. Doctors recommended operation to fit a pacemaker, which I could not afford. Further, doctors gave me a course of injections for about 8 months but the problems continued.. Lastly doctors told my husband to take me home for good as they felt no treatment other than fitting a pacemaker would help me. At that time, my husband attended Dr. Biswaroop Roy's Disease Reversal Seminar and immediately got me started on Wheatgrass. Within two months my heartbeat reached up to normal rate, my weight increased by 8 Kgs and my anemia problem was also solved.

ANEMIA
Sumeet Goyal (Male patient, Age 35 Yrs.), Mangalore

I was feeling run down and tired. I went to the doctor and they did some blood tests and found out that I was experiencing an extreme case of iron-deficiency anemia. The doctor gave me a prescription for strong iron pills. I had taken iron pills in the past. They made me nauseated and constipated. I was not interested in doing this, so I started to look for more natural ways to address the anemia.

I came to know about Wheatgrass benefits while attending Dr. Biswaroop Roy's Disease Reversal   Seminars. I decided to try drinking the Wheatgrass juice and I found great success.

When they first took my blood, it was way below the proper iron range. After 2 months of drinking wheatgrass juice, I was in the high numbers of the iron range.

For those two months, I drank wheatgrass juice shots, 3 times per week. Drinking the wheatgrass juice was the answer for me and it did not have any bad side effects!

OLD HABITS DIE HARD
Anju Datta (Female,Age 32 yrs), Noida

For years I have found it very difficult to try and do away with the standard "office drug"- tea & coffee and never succeeded until I took the Wheatgrass juice. Even then it came as a surprise-I never expected it to even do this, on the first day ! I am using it as part of sensible eating diet and it positively suppresses my food cravings which is ideal. I'm about 6 kgs s overweight and I've lost 2 kgs already. At last the ultimate Natural medicine has arrived. I only expect you to believe this once you have tried some."

INSOMNIA AND ANXIETY
Yogesh Saini (Male patient ,Age 42 yrs.), Jamshedpur

Due to extreme stress and overwork in the Office I had been loosing my sleep for quite a long time now. It started affecting my work badly. Then I met Dr. Biswaroop Roy who is 2 times Guinnesss World Record holder. He holds record not only for Fastest Memory but also for completing 198 pushups in just one minute. How could anyone maintain such a good health in todays fast paced overstressed overloaded life! He then revealed his secret to me. Now I am following his footsteps and regularly taking Wheatgrass juice two times a day. I have started feeling the difference. At the end of the day am as fresh as Dew and my sleeps are now uninterrupted and peaceful. Thanks to Dr Roy!!!

MENOPAUSAL PROBLEMS
Promila Bali (female patient, Age 50 Yrs.), Patiala

I am 50 years old and was having significant pre-menopausal symptoms for the past year. I talked to by GYN about it and tried several things which worked but which were really chemical in nature and not good for me. So, I started taking Wheatgrass juice and I have never felt better! The juice completely did away with all of my symptoms, from insomnia and irritability to hot flashes. In addition, I can tell that my body is just functioning better in general. The dark circles under my eyes which I have had to cover up for years are all clear, and my skin has never looked better. I have been on it now for about 3 months..

TOOTHACHE AND MOUTH ODOURS
Vishwajeet Bhatt (Male patient, Age 26 yrs), Delhi

I started wheatgrass juice as a part of my regular health maintainence as I am Health and body conscious person..But I observed that besides giving me a nutritious diet my tooth decaying process has stopped plus my foul mouth odours were gone without using mouth freshners...

GASTROINTESTINAL CONDITIONS
Pankaj Dhatwalia (Male patient, Age 34 yrs.), Bangalore

I have been suffering from various gastrointestinal problems due to my unhealthy eating habits. I attended Dr Biswaroop Seminars and found out about the Acid-Alkaline balance of the body. My eating habits had acidified my body and hence my gastrointestinal problems. Dr. Roy told me that I need to alkalize my body to regain my health and asked me to switch to Wheatgrass. As advised I have been taking Wheatgrass juice for four months now and it seems as if I have never been suffering from any disease at all...I feel hale and hearty as ever..All my problems disappeared but I continued drinking wheatgrass as it is very nutritious and keeps me energetic all day.

ULCERATIVE COLITIS
Poonam Jaiswal(Female patient, Age 31 yrs.), Agra

Colitis is very painful and I have been living with it for 5 yrs now..Am continuously on medicine but my condition never seems to improve..As an alternative cure I decided to try Wheatgrass. Wheatgrass proved to be very soothing and my burning sensation subsided within a month. I can now eat a wide variety of food without much problem. My colitis has reduced and I feel better now.

SMOKING
Babloo Vaidya (Male Patient, Age 27 Yrs.), Patna

I had been a chain smoker since I was five.I tried to quit smoking many times but failed. My health had deteriorated miserably. Then I attended Dr. Biswaroop's Behaviour Modification Seminars and came to know how to manage my cravings and how to modify my bad habit, and also came to know about the amazing benefits of Wheatgrass to claim my deteriorated health back. I am a regular Wheatrass juice drinker now.

My smoking habit is long gone and I feel as energetic as a racing horse...

CHAPTER -TWENTY FIVE

SECRETS OF
WORLD'S HEALTHIEST PEOPLE

Every person on this Earth wants to live forever, stay young and look beautiful forever. But, whatever our philosophy and thoughts about life are, there is undeniable, inevitable and ever-present fact, that each and every one of us is growing older. For many of us ageing is a source of grief and angst because old age is often, rather always, considered a synonym for deteriorating health, frailty, unattractive appearances and what not. We fear the curse of old age.

In the last 100 years we have added nearly 30 years to the average Life expectancy but the late years of life are not happy but pitiable, miserable and diseased. People live long but ironically fall sick repeatedly. In other words we have extended human life span but we have not extended the human health span.

But this is not true with all, people who have learnt to live in harmony with their body & natural force of life, things are different for them. There are cultures whose ways have stood the test of time that can stand on the path of wellness and joy. There is population of highly spirited, vigorous people who are healthy in their seventies, eighties and nineties. Their secrets have been corroborated and explained. It reveals that we all have tools to live longer and to remain active, productive and resourceful until the very end.

Let us read about some of the world's healthiest and most long living people and understand the key factors that influence human prospects for long and healthy life.

These are:

1. Abkhazia – Ancients of the Caucasus

2. Vilcabamba – The valley of eternal youth

3. Hunza – The people who dances in their nineties

4. The Centenarians of Okinawa

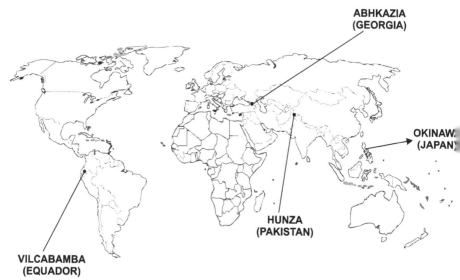

WORLD'S HEALTHIEST TRIBES

Abkhazia:

Abkhazia is an autonomous region within Soviet Georgia. Abkhazia covers three thousand square miles between the eastern shores of the Black sea and the Crestline of the main Caucasus range . It is bordered on the north by Russia and on the south by Georgia.

The Abkhazia are known for their extraordinary number of healthy centenarians (people who live above the age of 100 years). These people have maintained their vitality and strength to the very end of their long lives.

Their traditional diet is essentially vegetarian. Their breakfast usually consists of green vegetables freshly picked from the garden. During spring season it is made up of pungent vegetables such as watercress, green onions and radish. In summer and autumn tomatoes and cucumber are more popular .While winter salad consists of pickled cucumber, tomatoes, radish, cabbage and onion. At all three meals ,their people eat their beloved "abista", a cornmeal porridge, always freshly cooked and served warm. They eat fruits from their own orchards. There are cherries, apricots, pears, plums, peaches, figs, berries, grapes and apples. The fruit that is not eaten fresh is stored or dried for winter use. Freshly pickled and all vegetables are eaten raw or cooked in only a very small amount of water. Leftovers are discarded.

Nuts play a major role and form the fat diet. Almonds, pecans, beechnuts and hazelnuts cultivated form a part of everyday meal.

Abkhazians eat relatively less meat. They do not consume sugar, salt and butter.

On a whole Abkhazians consume proteins in moderate, fats mainly from nuts, carbohydrates from vegetables, fruits and whole grain cereals such as cornmeal abista.

Vilcabamba: The Valley of Eternal Youth

The second people famous for their longevity and health are the Vilcamambans. Vilcabamba is a small town in Ecuador's Ande's mountains, at an altitude of 4,500 feet and not far from Peruvian border.

This is a place where degenerative diseases seldom affect the population. The people have no heart disease, no caner, no diabetes, no stroke ,no cirrhosis, no sensitivity, no arteriosclerosis. The inhabitants of this place are able to live the full complement of mankind's years – more than a century.

Vilcamambans diet is almost entirely vegetarian, made up of whole grains, vegetables, fruits, seeds, beans and nuts. Their overall diet is very low in calories, so there are no overweight people in Vilcabamba.

Their protein comes from vegetables, whole grains and a variety of beans. Their carbohydrates are always unrefined and come primarily from whole grain cereals such as corn, quinoa, wheat and barley tubers including potatoes, yucca, sweet potatoes. Their fat comes from avocados seeds and nuts.

Hunza: People who dance in their nineties

Hunza lies at the northernmost tip of Pakistan, where Pakistan meets Russia and China. The people of Hunza live in an extraordinary fertile valley that has sustained a population of 10,000 to 30,000 people for 2000 years in complete isolation from rest of the world.

They grow up a wide variety of fruit including apricots, peaches, pears, apples, plums, grapes, cherries, mulberries & wild berries. In Hunza, the primary grains are wheat, barley, millet, buckwheat and the hard, pearly seeds of a grass called Job's tears.

Vegetables play a prominent role in the Hunzan diet and particularly greens – like mustard greens, spinach greens and lettuce and others like carrots, turnips, potatoes, radishes, beans, chickpeas, lentils and other sprouted legumes plus many kinds of pumpkins and other squashes. They grow flax meals which is used in almost every meal.

In Hunza, a large part of the diet is eaten uncooked. As much as 80% of the food is eaten in its natural state. Hunzan's soak lentils, beans and peas in water for several days then lay them out on wet clothes under the sun. They are eaten raw when they begin to sprout.

When vegetables are cooked they are lightly steamed using minimal amount of water and the water used to cook them is always consumed along with the vegetables.

In Hunza, Abkhazia & Vilcabamba a large proportion of elder citizens have remained vigorous and enjoyed life right up until their deaths. It is an established fact that the elderly in each of these regions have had extremely low rates of heart disease, cancer obesity, arthritis, asthma, dementia and the other degenerative infirmities that plague so many older people around the globe.

The Centenarians of Okinawa

The southmost Japenese state of Okinawa is made up of 161 beautiful islands that are the dwelling place of 1.4 million people. This place is blessed with an abundance of flora and fauna, pristine rain forest. For most of the people, Okinawa is known, being home for the largest American military presence in the far East as well as for having been the site of the longest and bloodiest battle of World War II.

Recently Okinawa has became known to be the home of the longest living and healthiest people ever, throughly studied.

Researchers tell that it is a normal occurrence in Okinawa to find energetic great grandfathers living in their own homes, tending their own gardens and on weekends being visited by their grandchildren, who would qualify for senior citizens. It is a common place for people in Okinawa to live past the age of 100 and remain active ,healthy and youthful looking. If you ask elder Okinawans for the key to their legendary health and longevity they simply point to the nutritious and wholesome food they eat.

Okinawans diet is 20% lower in calories than the Japanese average and contains 300% of the green/yellow vegetables, particularly high on sweet potatoes.The Okinawans diet is low in fat and 75% of the grains of the average Japanese dietary intake. It also includes small amount of fish and more of soy and legumes.

The Okinawans almost never over-eat and follow the following two diet rules :-
Rule I - Eat to 80% full.

Rule II – Eat healthy foods, mostly plants.

In 1951, Okinawa legally became a possession of the United States and the U.S. Military till 1972.The massive American presence had a mammoth impact on the culture and lifestyle in Okinawa. With the American soldiers came American fast-food Restaurants. MacDonalds, KFC, Burgerking and Baskin&Robbins have become a commonplace. Okinawa now has more hamburger restaurants than anywhere else in Japan. As a result of these influences, younger Okinawan's are eating processed food, meat, sugar, corn syrup, and burger and pizza. The elder Okinawans, whose health and longevity have been documented so thoroughly, eat a diet that is plant based and low calorie. But their younger generations fill their shopping carts with all types of processed food.

Today, Okinawans in their forties and fifties are increasingly overweight and are more likely to die of heart attacks. They have the highest level of obesity in Japan, the worst cardiovascular risk profile, highest risk of coronary heart disease and the highest risk for premature death.

In Okinawa today we can see both, an ultimate example of healthful living and its opposite within the same gene pool, and both taking place at a time when they can be studied carefully by scientific investigators.

We can see that the Diets of the World's exceptionally healthy and long lived people have a great deal in common:
i) They are all low in overall calories.
ii) They are all high in good carbohydrates including plenty of whole grains, vegetables and fruits.
iii) They all depend on fresh foods ,eating primarily what is in season, locally grown rather than relying on canned foods.
iv) They are all low in fat and the fat comes from natual sources, including seeds, nuts in some cases fish and not from bottled oils, margarines etc.
v) They derive their proteins primarily from plant sources including

beans, peas, whole grains, seeds and nuts.

vi) They drink a lot of green leafy vegetable juices like spinach, barley and Wheatgrass.

THE TRADITIONAL DIETS OF THESE LONG-LIVED CULTURES ARE REMARKABLY SIMILAR

	Abkhazia	Vilcabmba	Hunza	Okinawa
Percent of calories from carbohydrates	65%	74%	73%	72%
Percent of calories from fat	20%	15%	17%	18%
Percent of calories from protein	15%	11%	10%	10%
Overall daily calories (adult males)	1,900	1,800	1,900	1,900
Percentage of diet from plant foods	90%	99%	99%	94%
Percentage of diet from animal foods	10%	1%	1%	6%
Salt consumption	low	low	low	low
Sugar consumption	0	0	0	0
Processed food consumption: 0	0	0	0	
Incidence of obesity	0	0	0	0

In November 2005 National Geographic published a cover story titled 'The Secrets of Living Longer'. The lead article featured 3 contemporary groups of long living people, those from Okinawa – Japan, Sardini – Italy & Loma Linda-California, all of whom eat a plant based diet. At the conclusion of the issue, National Geographic summarised the 'Secrets of Long Life' in two words 'GO VEGETARIAN'.

CHAPTER -TWENTY SIX

MEDIA COMMENT ON WHEATGRASS

	Comments
The New York Times Expect the World® January 4, 1998	'Wheatgrass... kind of cleans out your system and opens up your oxygen pores,"........
The Seattle Times October 6, 2009	For true believers, wheatgrass is the Holy Grail of Nutrition, it washes drug deposits from the body, neutralizes toxins, purifies the liver and prevents tooth decay.....
abcNEWS Aug. 10, 2011	Wheatgrass cleanses the body and slows the aging process
Los Angeles Times June 16, 2003	It prevents cavities, lowers cholesterol, heals wounds, stops hair from graying, aids digestion and cures cancer.........
TIME July 22, 1940	Chlorophyll treatment had been used in 1,200 cases of infection, ranging from peritonitis to pyorrhea and the common cold. For lung and brain abscesses, abdominal infections like peritonitis, a solution of chlorophyll in salt water was applied directly to the infected surfaces, either in wet dressings or through soft rubber tubes. "Indolent" ulcers and "weeping" skin diseases were treated with a paste of chlorophyll.....

BBC NEWS Tuesday, 10 April 2007	Wheatgrass is packed with so many nutrients that they are particularly good for our health...
planet green Tue Dec 30, 2008	• Wheatgrass a powerful detoxifier (i.e., hangover cure) • It has been used successfully to treat peptic ulcers, ulcerative colitis, constipation, diarrhea, and other gastrointestinal issues.
THE ASIAN AGE Jun 20, 2010	Wheatgrass provides the much needed nutrients and minerals to the body, besides supplying a good quantity of vitamin E, iron and vitamins of the vitamin B group.
The Statesman 14 May 2011	As regular blood transfusions were not only painful but also expensive, Dr. Mukherjee advised Ashim to give Moinam Wheat grass juice as it reduced transfusion requirement in patients with Thalassemia...
the pioneer June 22, 2011	Wheatgrass is a power packed booster with various nutrients and minerals.....and helps controlling diabetes besides other ailments.

DECCAN HERALD May 05, 2006	Wheatgrass, an organic powerhouse of amino acids, vitamins, minerals and chlorophyll, cleanses the digestive system and removes toxins. It is easily digested and absorbed and enhances immunity. Did you know that 1 oz of wheatgrass juice contains the nutritional equivalent of 2.5 lbs of leafy, green vegetables!
Chronicle DECCAN June 23, 2011	Depleted soil conditions and refining give us nutritionally bankrupt foods which fill us without nourishing us. This leads to constant hunger at the cellular level. Solution: Turn to "superfood" Wheatgrass to satisfy your 'cellular' hunger. Voila! You will eat less and feel more satisfied without dieting!
THE HINDU May 01, 2005	Wheatgrass is full of good stuff. Wheatgrass helps maintain good health and fight ailments like asthma, inflammation and arthritis. Wheatgrass, or its juice, helps fight many chronic ailments — from simple anaemia to leukaemia, from skin rash to cancer, from worms to ulcers.
THE TIMES OF INDIA Feb 5, 2009	It was in 2006 that the scientists from NRS Medical College, Netaji Subhas Cancer Research Institute (NSCRI) and Central Ayurvedic Drug Research got together to analyze the properties of Wheat grass.

HindustanTimes July 21, 2011	Metal and chemical toxins add to adrenal fatigue:Detoxify your body by having at least two glasses of *Wheatgrass*........ Wheatgrass Juice: This is a miraculous juice for those suffering from hypertension, as it is a rich source of magnesium and potassium. Both minerals can lower blood pressure. Getting enough magnesium and potassium can also lessen the dosage of medicine you are consuming.
Chandigarh **Tribune** Chandigarh, June 26	For many Thalassaemic patients, who require units of blood after every few weeks, wheatgrass proving nothing less than a panacea......
The Tribune Sunday, January 7, 2001	Wheat grass juice: A miracle on earth, the most vital ingredient in wheatgrass is chlorophyll. It is contained in chloroplast that produces nutritious elements with the help of sunlight. Therefore, in the words of Dr. Burshar, a scientist, it is a concentrated solar energy. Though this substance exists in all green plants but wheat grass is perhaps the best source for obtaining chlorophyll.

CHAPTER -TWENTY SEVEN

REFERENCES FROM MEDICAL JOURNALS

Journal / University / Researcher center	Reference
http://tuh.templehealth.org/ content/default.htm# **Temple University**	In more than 1,000 cases treated at Temple University Hospital by Drs. Robert Ferguson Ridpath and Thomas Carroll Davis, there was "not a single case recorded in which either improvement or cure . . . [did] not take place."
UTHealth The University of Texas Health Science Center at Houston **Texas Medical Center** An Orginization of Non-Profit Healthcare Providers	In 1980, Dr. Chiu Nan Lai at the University of Texas Medical Center, reported that extracts of wheat grass and other green vegetables inhibit the cancer-causing effects of two mutagens (benzopyrene and methylcholanthrene). The more chlorophyll in the vegetable, the greater the protection from the carcinogen
MSNJ MEDICAL SOCIETY OF NEW JERSEY	Dr. S. A. Chernomosky, in a 1988 review article in the New Jersey Medical Journal, states that the treatment of patients with slow-healing wounds is still problematic, and that the increased use of chlorophyll compounds may offer a useful alternative in this area....

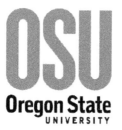 **Oregon State** UNIVERSITY	Chlorophyllin has been used orally as an internal deodorant and topically in the treatment of slow-healing wounds for more than 50 years without any side effects. Chlorophylls and chlorophyllin form molecular complexes with some chemicals known or suspected to cause cancer, and in doing so, may block carcinogenic effects. Carefully controlled studies have not been undertaken to determine whether a similar mechanism might limit uptake of required nutrients.
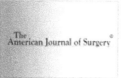 The American Journal of Surgery	Gruskin, B. 1940. Chlorophyll — its therapeutic place in acute and suppurative disease Collings, G. 1945. Chlorophyll of wheat grass extract in the local treatment of burns. American Journal of Surgery 70:58-63.
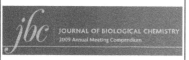 **JOURNAL OF BIOLOGICAL CHEMISTRY** 2009 Annual Meeting Compendium	Kohler, G. 1944. The effect of stages of growth on the chemistry of the grasses. Kohler, G. 1939. Relation of pyrrole-containing pigments to hemoglobin synthesis. Journal of Biological Chemistry. 128:501-509. Kohler, G., Randle, S. and Wagner, J. 1939. The Grass Juice Factor.

The Japanese Journal of **PHARMACOLOGY** The Japanese Pharmacological Society	Nagai, H. Nishiyori, T. Daikoku, M. and Koda, A. 1983. Immunopharmacological studies of sodium copper chlorophyllin.
ARCHIVES INTERNAL MEDICINE	Patek, A. 1936. Chlorophyll and regeneration of the blood.
New York State journal of medicine New York State Medical Association	120. Sack, P., and Barnard, R. 1955. Studies on the hemagglutinating and inflammation properties of exudate from nonhealing wounds and their inhibition by chlorophyll derivatives. October 15, 1955, p.2952-2956.
The Journal of Physiology A publication of The Physiological Society	Hughes, J. and Latner, A. 1936. Wheat grass and haemoglobin regeneration after haemorrhage.

CHAPTER –TWENTY EIGHT

CELEBRITY WHEATGRASS USERS

LANCE ARMSTRONG

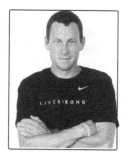

Lance Edward Armstrong (born on September 18, 1971) is an American former professional road racing cyclist who won the Tour de France, a record seven consecutive times, after having survived testicular cancer. He is also the founder and chairman of the Lance Armstrong Foundation for cancer research and support. He last rode for (and helped found) UCI Pro Team Team Radio Shack.

In October 1996 he was diagnosed as having testicular cancer, a tumor that had spread to his brain and lungs. His cancer treatments included brain and testicular surgery and extensive chemotherapy, and his prognosis was originally poor. He then resorted to wheatgrass juice and recovered soon. He was back on the track and went on to win Tour de France each year from 1999 to 2005, and is the only person to win seven times, having broken the previous record of five wins.

BILL CLINTON 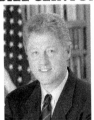	The former U.S. president who was once known for his love for barbecue, MacDonald's, KFC has radically changed his diet in an effort to combat his heart disease. His new vegan food diet now includes wheatgrass juice everyday.
BACKSTREET BOYS 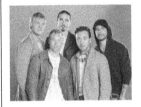	**Backstreet Boys** (sometimes referred to as **BSB**) are an American vocal group. They rose to fame with their debut international album, *Backstreet Boys* (1996). They rose to superstardom with their album *Millennium* (1999) and its follow-up album, *Black & Blue* (2000). Backstreet Boys always take a shot of wheatgrass juice before going on stage, because they say it gives them energy boost and helps them perform better.
KATE MOSS 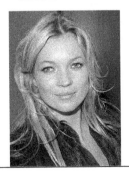	**Kate Moss** is an English supermodel. Moss is known for her waifish figure and popularising the heroin chic look in the 1990s, which made her a supermodel. She is also known for her controversial private life, high profile relationships, party lifestyle, and drug use. To adopt a healthy lifestyle she decided to start with wheatgrass juice. She consumes wheatgrass in the morning as well as in the evenings.

ELIZABETH HURLEY 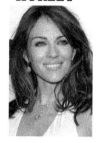	Elizabeth Hurley is an English model and actress, best known for her long-standing career modeling for Estée Lauder perfumes. To keep her figure petite, she follows a strict regime of daily yoga, and wheatgrass juice everyday.
GWYNETH PALTROW 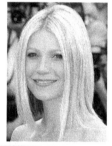	**Gwyneth Kate Paltrow** is an American actress and singer. She made her acting debut on stage in 1990 and started appearing in films in 1991. **Gwyneth Paltrow** is not a fan of moderation. She's uses wheatgrass juice to detox her body after a night of hard party.
ANGELINA JOLIE 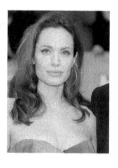	Angelina Jolie is an American actress and was named Hollywood's highest-paid actress by Forbes in 2009 and 2011. Jolie is noted for promoting humanitarian causes as a Goodwill Ambassador for the United Nations High Commissioner for Refugees (UNHCR. Angelina Jolie during her pregnancy drank wheatgrass juice everyday. After delivering the baby she drank wheatgrass juice religiously to get back into her shape.

CHAPTER -TWENTY NINE

DOCTOR'S COMMENTS

Wheatgrass juice is a god gift in the arena of lifestyle diseases.Now no killer cardiac attacks or diabetes or depression.I can say rog anek dawa ek.....Wheatgrass.!

Dr Roop Singh MBBS, MD(General Medicine) Best Doctor Award Winner IMA 2006, Jaipur

Wheat Grass is the green blood, which purifies our red blood and white blood cells and cures us from many diseases including life threatening diseases like cancer and hepatitis. I am among one of the testimonials having cured myself from cancer and hepatitis-C. Dr Biswaroop Roy Chowdhury always shows us the shortest way of long lasting healthy and happy life through natural way by blending diet of soul (positive thoughts) and diet of body (green blood). His book - "Heal Without Pill" - is a must read book.

Dr. BK Chandra Shekhar, Author of 'Invisible Doctor' and a Cancer Survivor, Faridabad

Processed food and fast food are curse on our society. They should be completely done away. Most of the diseases are born out of these. Healthy and nutritious food habits should be inculcated. This books is an eye opener for any layman

Dr Ashok Mehta, FRCS, BC Roy Award Winner, Medical Director, BSESMG Hospital, Mumbai

This book is complete in itself. Its raises questions on today's food habits, takes a journey to the healthiest habits, gives references from medical studies and researches and then provides answers to all the questions satisfactorily. Nice work done by Biswaroop.

Dr S Viswanathan, FRCS, Director (Centre for Yoga Studies, Annamalai Univercity), Medical Superintendent, RMCMS, Chidambaram

The book is awesome....new concepts...I myself have learnt a lot from the book with the surety of a complete health.....an eye opener.

Dr. Reena Tomar, MBBS, MD. Pathology
AIIMS, New Delhi

India being the world capital of diabetes and all diabetic being heart patient, if they go no tobacco, no non – vegetarian and only Naturopathic food, we can prevent silent heart attacks as recommended in the book of Biswaroop Roy Chowdhury.

Dr. Siddharth, Cardiologist,
Medicity Medanta, Gurgaon

I feel strongly that vitamin B-12 and Folate are must for mental wellness. By diet improvement and changes in life style and including wheat grass juice in routine as suggested by writer of the book, can guaranteed prevention of the degeneration of brain and thus causing depression.

Dr. Puneet, Psychiatrist,
Max Hospital, New Delhi

Stress causes acidity, ulcer even gut Bleeding in adrenaline junkies. People who are always tensed, produce adrenaline. Wheat grass juice, can produce anti stress hormones for them.

Dr. Meer Kausari, Gastro – Enterologist
Artemis Hospital, Gurgaon

By going through contents of Biswaroop Roy Chowdhury's book, I am thrilled that a neuron and brain centre can be stimulated by methods suggested in the book.

Dr. Kapil Agrwal, M.D. Neurology
Paras Hospital, Gurgaon

Every now and then you read a book which is so inspiring and such a pleasure that you feel impelled to read further, finish and walk on the street shouting "read this!" Well, I've just read Dr. Biswaroop Roy Chowdhury's book and I urge everyone to buy or borrow a copy without a delay.

Dr. Mahendra N.Kabra, M.D.(Hom), Doctor of The Year 2010
Research Award from World Congress 1996' for Vitiligo
Swami Vivekanand Yuva Gaurav iin "Scientist Category"

The chief aim & main thrust of the book is to ensure physical, mental, psychological, emotional development & well being of human being. BOOK is simply GREAT. ...

Dr. Sharad Bhatt (Rtd lt. Colnel, Bsc, BDS KGMC, Lko GMP, IIM Lko)
Ex JOINT DIRECTOR Dental Services, GOI

This book is really an" Eye Opener" as you mentioned rightly even for me though, I am working as Corporate Health Consultant having 15 years of experience in the field of Preventive Health. Its really a new beginning for every one who reads and practices consistently and with dedication. The separate tabulation mentioning Acid and Alkali food is really fantastic. The Testimonials and success stories are really motivating and mind blowing.

Dr. Remya Mahesh MBBS, AFIH, DHA, Corporate Health
Consultant, Lokmanya Hospital, PUNE

Biswaroop Intelligent Food Theory is amazing. Information on MSG and ASPARTAME is quite enlightening and an eye opener. Since then I have stopped eating outside food. Now my food mostly comprises of natural raw food. I have even started wheatgrass therapy and have started growing wheatgrass myself....Am going to propagate it intensively.

Dr. Jagdeesh, B.D. S, Udupi, Karnatka

"Heal Without Pill"....is a must read. Every chapter in the book is "Food for thought".

Dr. Dana Azim, Clinical Psychologist, Chennai

The intricate balance between various dietary factors can be mind boggling for any common man but are true to the core. Understanding and balancing these should be done in a natural way as propagated by Dr. Biswaroop Roy Chowdhury.

Dr. Sujata Rathi, Dietician, GHRC, Mt Abu

Behavior Modification Theory and BRAIN as explained by the book is easily comprehendible and achievable. Useful for everyone in today's stressful world.

Dr. Namrata, BSES Hospital, Mumbai

Wheatgrass seems to be a complete food in itself! Very interesting.

Dr. Ankita, MD, Ahmadabad

Various studies on Wheatgrass Therapy and references from medical journals establishes wheatgrass as a cure and opens up new avenues for complementary medicines.

Dr. Sachin Parab, MD (Medicine), Thane, Mumbai

Wheatgrass has all the potential to emerge as a powerful cure and source of nutrition. More extensive research into it will benefit mankind immensely.

Dr. Shubdha Neel, Neel Hospital, Panvel, Navi Mumbai

World's healthiest tribes were an interesting read. There is no substitute for 'Raw Fruits and Vegetables'. Biswaroop's effort to promote raw food is commendable. Parents should take a note of this.

Dr. Punit Saxena, MD, Surat

Wheatgrass has a long way to go. Researches done in this field prove this. Though more effort should be done to back it up as a total cure.

Dr. Ganesh, MD, Ahmedabad

An illustrated book with easy to learn remedies that, perhaps even our ancestors used for curing their diseases. It is just like Ayurveda that uses herbs like tulsi and amla to cure diseases. It also tells us how to prevent common diseases like cold and cough. Every person of any age must read this book for this is how you eradicate diseases and live a life longer and healthier than before. In one word it can be said that this book is very ENLIGHTENING.

Dr. R.S. Mehra, M.B.B.S., Surat

This is a 'must read' for all who intend to live a long and healthy life. Nature is indeed self sufficient . Healing capacities of it were undermined, till I read this book and my views on nature as a great healer are reassured and strengthened. Jaw drooping facts complied in the book are really an eye opener. Panacea of all ailments on earth is 'go vegetarian'. I prescribe this book to all.

Dr. Pankaj Sharma, M.B.A (Hospital Administration), New Delhi

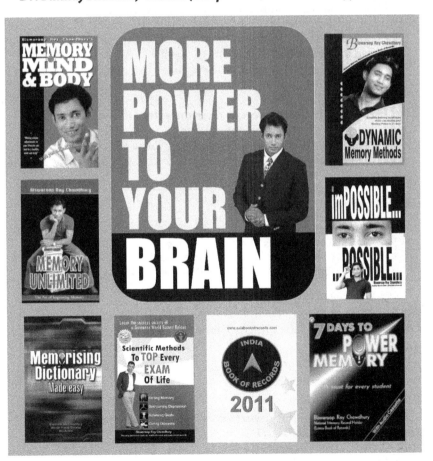

CHAPTER -THIRTY

LAST BUT NOT THE LEAST

By now you must be completely convinced and accredited the fact that wheat grass is a wonderful plant. It would not be an exaggeration if I call it as '**Kamdenu**'.

I would like to share a few very common and oft repeated queries about wheat grass

1) Why is Wheatgrass not popular among masses and is not even marketed by pharmaceuticals company in spite of numerous health benefits?

Ans) This is because Wheatgrass, in natural form, cannot be patented and Pharmaceutical companies don't sell products that cannot be patented. Another major commercial reason is that if Wheatgrass is readily available and makes people healthy, then who will buy their expensive, complicated, dead medicines!

not to miss, even today this is being used by people in remote areas of our country, where advance treatments and hospitals are still unavailable

2) How effective is powdered wheatgrass and Wheatgrass pills?

Ans) Wheatgrass is effective when consumed fresh within 20 mins of its juicing. Pills and powdered Wheatgrass loose most of its nutrient - value in process. Consuming them like consuming dry, powdered wood!

Contact us for:
1. In House Mind-Body Workshop.
2. Health SMS Services.
3. Certified Wheatgrass Therapist training..
4. Installation of Super Specialty Home Hospital.
5. Products related to Super Specialty Home Hospital.
6. Books and CD's
7. Opening your own Wheatgrass centre.

Tele fax: +91- 0129-2510534
Phone: +91-9312286540 (10am to 5pm, Sunday Closed).

Address: Dynamic Memory Pvt. Ltd.
B- 121, 2nd Floor, Green Fields, Faridabad-121003 Haryana (India)

Website: www.biswaroop.com

E-mail: biswaroop@yahoo.com

Like us on facebook:http://www.facebook.com/pages/Biswaroop-Roy-Chowdhury/117044468312071

CPSIA information can be obtained
at www.ICGtesting.com
Printed in the USA
FSHW021953291021
85864FS